CONQUERING
AUTISM

CONQUERING AUTISM

Reclaiming Your Child
Through Natural Therapies

◆

STEPHEN B. EDELSON, M.D.

TWIN STREAMS
KENSINGTON PUBLISHING CORP.
http://www.kensingtonbooks.com

TWIN STREAM BOOKS are published by

Kensington Publishing Corp.
850 Third Avenue
New York, NY 10022

ISBN 0-7582-0184-2

First Hardcover Printing: April 2003
First Trade Paperback Printing: January 2004
10   9   8   7   6   5   4   3   2

Printed in the United States of America

This book is dedicated to my wife, Carol, who has always been the major supporting structure in my endeavor to achieve the best in the work that I do. And to my children, Dana, Richard, Alex, Brad, and Joshua, who make me want to continue to produce. Lastly, to my mother and deceased father who were there from the beginning.

Acknowledgments

I wish to thank M. Nathaniel Mead and Sarah Fremerman for their word-smithing and research expertise, and for guiding me through the various stages of this book's birthing process. I offer my heartfelt thanks to David Cantor, Ph.D., for his help in the statistical analyses we used in our peer-reviewed medical articles. I am also indebted to the Edelson Center staff, which includes my clinical supervisor, Danna Carlson and my front office manager, Maria Speizer. Over the last two years, there have been many other employees at the Center, and I would like to thank all of them for their dedicated assistance in running it. For critical assistance in laboratory diagnostic assessments of immunocompetence, immunotoxicology profiles, oxidative stress profiles, and other relevant aspects of physiological integrity, I would like to thank the following individuals and diagnostic laboratories: Aristo Vojdani, Ph.D., of Immunosciences Lab, Inc. (Beverly Hills, CA); Great Smokies Diagnostic Laboratories (Asheville, NC); John L. Lasseter, Ph.D., of Accu-Chem Laboratories (Richardson, TX); and Jonathan Pangborn, Ph.D. of Bionostics (St. Charles, IL). I am grateful to Kensington editors Elaine Sparber and Jeremie Ruby-Strauss, for their editing and steadfast guidance, and to Lee Heiman, for giving me the opportunity to write this book. Thanks also goes to Mari Florence, publisher of Really Great Books in Los Angeles, for her creative thoughts and efforts to help launch the project. Lastly, I wish to express my gratitude to all the parents who asked me to care for their children over the years. Without their hope and courage, I could not have unveiled the deeper levels of biological disorder that underlie the disease we call autism.

Contents

Preface

The human brain is a marvelous creation through which all our feelings, thoughts, and actions are formed. Our central nervous system is so intricately designed that even subtle changes in brain function can profoundly influence those feelings, thoughts, and actions. In autistic children, however, these changes are far from subtle. My own research suggests that the changes that occur in autistic brains have their roots in environmental toxicities that have become all but ubiquitous in our modern world.

We now know that drugs, pesticides, solvents, heavy metals, and other insidious forms of environmental pollution can dramatically affect brain function throughout life. But the human brain is particularly vulnerable during pre- and postnatal development, and the sources of toxic insult are often, sadly, a crapshoot—toxins released from fatty tissues of the mother, from her dental amalgams, or from vapors inadvertently inhaled at the workplace. We have had the opportunity to study the mothers of autistic children, and they always have the same toxic characteristics as the infected child. The placenta and the breast are the avenues for transmission of these toxins. My research, published in peer-reviewed scientific journals, suggests that the key to unlocking the secret of autism lies in understanding the ecological factors that damage the brain in this early-life period.

Pediatricians and other professionals who work in the area of children's mental health can no longer understand the fundamental biology of the developing brain without also studying the impact of neurotoxins during early life and the vital importance of the body's own detoxication mechanisms. What is equally true is that parents of children with autistic brains cannot fully understand their son or daughter without learning about the factors needed to keep this aberrant brain protected from toxic insults.

For me, this awakening was spawned in the early 1990s, as I began to redirect my clinical research energies toward understanding the roots of autism. My training in family medicine had taught me to think globally and innovatively about the problems I was confronting in daily clinical practice. During the 1990s, I saw more and more children not just with autism, but neurodevelopmental deficits in general. Although I had culti- vated a keen interest in this area, the science had always seemed shaky at best. As we entered the 1990s, however, an explosion of interest in brain research helped the medical community garner a clearer understanding of the behavioral and cognitive impacts of chemical changes in the infant brain. This explosion coincided with a sudden surge in environmental medi- cine research, a surge fueled largely by the convergence of three disci- plines: neurobiology, immunotoxicology, and behavioral medicine.

Suddenly, the scientific underpinnings of neurodevelopmental disor- ders had solidified to the extent that I could begin to assemble the autistic puzzle. This book represents the culmination of those efforts. It was con- ceived to explain not just the "why" of autism, but also the "how" and "what" of autistic treatment. It provides a logical, practical foundation for liberating young children—as much as is biologically feasible—from the seemingly intractable confines of the autistic mind.

If physicians, therapists, and researchers do not look below the surface to understand the underlying causes for autistic disorders, then behavioral interventions will provide only limited benefits. Unless the biological roots of this neurodevelopmental disorder are addressed as part of preven- tion and therapy, the behavioral, cognitive, emotional, social, and family problems will not improve. There is currently an epidemic of the autistic spectrum in all developed countries, and the rate is increasing. Society as a whole will continue to suffer under the growing burden of younger gen- erations who find it increasingly difficult to function normally in this world.

In the pages that follow I will explore many dimensions to the autistic problem, providing a considerable amount of investigative detail as well as practical tips and insights regarding the therapeutic process. I will address the main benefits of my biologically based program, as well as the chal- lenges that autistic children are likely to encounter as they undergo detox- ification and other vital strategies that are part and parcel of the Edelson treatment program. You will learn ways to make the program practical for your child, and you will learn the things that you can do at home, versus those that require the expertise of a skilled environmental physician.

My hope is that physicians around the country will take this book and begin to apply its basic teachings. It will offer appropriate guidelines to help parents and their autistic children move beyond the usually limited results that can be achieved with behavior modification strategies alone. With this basic information, parents and physicians can join together to forge a new alliance, one grounded in the principles of environmental medicine. Parents must assume a major role in reclaiming much of the inner life that has been stolen away from the autistic child. My clinical experience indicates that even the extremely autistic child can be helped—in many cases, dramatically—as long as they are still young, ideally—but not necessarily—between the ages of two and four. The journey is often a difficult one, but for everyone concerned, it is a journey that must be taken in order for deeper levels of healing to occur.

I rejoice whenever I see an autistic child undergo a dramatic transformation in their ability to function, think, and behave in ways that clearly reflect a definite degree of social awareness. I rejoice whenever I see a child once labeled autistic now playfully interacting with other children. I rejoice whenever such children smile at their parents, whenever I see them hugging their family members and expressing love. It is as if these children have emerged from their tunnel of silence and discovered life anew. It is as if these children have recovered something truly sacred about the human condition: the freedom of thought, feeling, and behavior that is everyone's birthright.

STEPHEN B. EDELSON, M.D.

CONQUERING
AUTISM

Chapter 1

◆

You Can Reverse Autism

We stand in the midst of an ominous epidemic, one that has claimed the minds of hundreds of thousands of young children. The incidence of the severe behavioral disorder known as autism, or *mindblindness,* has been increasing, and now surpasses both childhood cancer and Down syndrome. To date, there has been little relief for those who continue to suffer from the diverse range of disorders that fall within the *so-*called "autistic spectrum." Medical science has offered no definitive answer to this frightening problem.

In this book I present an answer, based on scientifically valid and often profound clinical experiences. The research conducted at our Atlanta-based clinic, now published in peer-reviewed medical journals, suggests that my multifaceted approach may be the most comprehensive and effective program for treating autism offered anywhere in the world.

At this writing I have treated and observed well over 200 young children diagnosed with autism. What I've learned from this experience is that a diagnosis of autism need not translate into a devastating life sentence. While the number of autistic children diagnosed each year continues to increase, there is light at the end of the tunnel. Autism is not only manageable, but in some cases ultimately reversible, or even curable.

My experience with treating this disease began in 1994. At that time, I began to explore novel strategies for bolstering the autistic body's ability to eliminate toxins. Since that time, I have worked with dozens of infants who never smiled or reached out to their parents. Toddlers who could walk, but who balked at human contact and recoiled from human touch as if from an electric shock. School-age children who disrupted entire class-rooms with tantrums or vocalizations that were more like shrieks than human speech. Children who evidently could not interpret facial expressions or emotions. Children who didn't know how to share or make friends, much less keep them. Children who fixated for hours on a doorknob, seemingly oblivious to the world around them. Children who seemed lost beyond measure.

Feelings of despair and helplessness are common among families with autistic children. Part of the problem is that no established medical treatment exists for autism. Therapists teach autistic children behavior modification techniques with varying success (though as I discuss later, most of this success is superficial, as many of the robot-like tendencies of autistic behavior remain). Medications have been tried to control the sometimes bizarre behavior of autistic children, but most drugs are not used because of ineffectiveness and major side effects.

Out of a combination of desperation and love for their children, millions of parents have tried everything short of witchcraft and psychic surgery to get their children back. They have begun placing their children on special diets, giving them dozens of supplements each day. The children will invariably undergo speech therapy and behavioral therapy. In time, if they seem stable enough, these children will head off to special ed classes at the local elementary school.

In many cases, children exposed to this scattershot approach will show incremental improvements over time. But without understanding the underlying cause of autism, the results are usually either very limited or short-lived. Many parents and physicians are still groping in the dark for a solution to this cruel illness.

Our First Study Uncovers the Toxic Connection

My initial research on autism grew out of my interest in the impact of the environment on the immune system. As I will show you later in this book, the immune-toxin link has provided many profound insights into a wide variety of diseases. The more we pollute the environment, the more damage we do to the immune system and the more this system tends to compromise the very body organs and systems it is designed to protect.

First, let me state the obvious—there's no question that autistic children have suffered some form of injury to the immune system, resulting in abnormal immune functioning. Many experts in the field of autism research have voiced this same basic truth.[1] What seems most striking is the fact that toxic chemicals and heavy metals such as mercury can produce the same kind of damaged immune system profile that has been seen in these children. Now, although I'm only theorizing that the pattern of immune dysfunction in these children results from toxic exposures, I do have some good research to back me up.

One form of immune dysfunction that reflects the adverse impact of the environment on health is that of allergy. In the fall of 1994, I viewed a videotape of a colleague interviewing the parents of his autistic patients. Intriguingly, all of these children had allergies, although there was no consistent pattern as to which allergies would develop. This basic observation suggested to me that something might be stressing the immune systems of these children, resulting in both a broad-spectrum allergic reactivity and brain injury at the same time.

My first study dealt not only with immunological and toxicological parameters, but also with nutritional biochemistry, the gastrointestinal system, neurotransmitter levels, liver detoxication (*detoxication* is the body's internal means of removing toxins, whereas *detoxification* refers to treatments or interventions aimed at stimulating the body's capacity to neutralize and/or eliminate toxins), and the vaccine issue (the combined vaccine for protection against measles, mumps, and rubella has been linked with autism). We performed a number of biochemical, immunological, and toxicological studies on them as part of our assessment process. Here's an overview of the tests we performed for this initial study:

- **Hair analysis and heavy metal challenge.** These tests measure the levels of heavy metals such as mercury and lead in the body. We wanted to find out if there was any relationship between the presence of these metals and autism, and to determine whether there was a way to remove these toxins.

- **Intestinal permeability.** This test tells us whether there is damage to the intestinal lining, which can allow toxins to "leak" into the body. It is important to find out if such damage has occurred, since the intestinal lining can be healed.

- **Glucaric acid and mercapturic acid.** These two tests tell us something about the burden of neurotoxic chemicals in the body. Toxic xenobiotic substances induce the activities of certain enzymes, which lead to the formation of glucaric acid. Measuring levels of this substance can help tell us something about how much stress the liver is under to detoxify such substances. Mercapturic acid levels directly reflect the degree or rate of detoxication of many foreign chemicals, including insecticides, herbicides, and fungicides, which are conjugated with glutathione to produce mercapturic acid. (Nicotine and caffeine can also contribute to elevations in mercapturic acid, but none of the patients in our study had a history of nicotine or caffeine use.)

• **Comprehensive stool analysis.** This test, which looks at the pathological ecology of the colon, can also help us detect problems related to a damaged intestinal lining. This area of study is particularly intriguing since much has been written on the relationship between poor digestion or malabsorption and infection in chronic illness.

• **Neurotransmitters.** Measuring the levels of neurotransmitters in blood platelets and urine helps us determine whether there is a deficiency caused by lack of neurotransmitter production or renal loss. This allows us to supplement the body with their precursors, and heal the abnormal renal process if necessary.

• **Candida immune complex and antigen levels.** This test shows levels of antigens (foreign proteins) and immune complexes (combinations of antibodies and antigens) in the blood, and indirectly reflects the burden of candida yeast infection the body.

• **Immune mechanisms.** The immunologic tests enable us to assess various aspects of immune system functioning and are also used to determine whether previous studies in this area were correct. The answers to these questions could lead us to a better understanding of the possible mechanism of damage in the brain in autistic children—for example, antimyelin antibody relationship. The tests we do here include the following: mitogen lymphocyte stimulation, T-cell subsets, IL-1 generation, autoantibody profile, chemical antibodies, immune complex formation, and vaccine antibodies.

• **Nutritional studies.** We evaluate vitamins, minerals, essential fatty acids, and amino acids, which gives us evidence of basic biochemical insufficiencies that are thought to be related to autism in its various forms.

• **Liver detoxication evaluation.** This study allows us to see whether the liver is working efficiently.

• **Toxic chemical blood levels.** This gives us evidence for a body burden of possibly neurotoxic chemicals.

• **Intradermal skin testing.** We use these tests to see if patients have activated immune systems and are sensitive to foods, chemicals, and other substances. Food and other allergies may be responsible for many autistic symptoms.

Using these tests in my initial study, what exactly did I find? The bodies of the first thirty children I examined showed very high levels of chemical toxins and heavy metals such as mercury, tin, and lead—all toxic to the nervous system. These children were far more burdened than other children their age. This led me to suspect that some of these toxins were a major factor in the development of autism and, possibly, other neurological problems in children.

After carefully studying the children with respect to all these characteristics, I gained a number of important insights about autism. About 25% of these children had an overgrowth of the yeast, *Candida albicans,* in their stools. At least half (50%) of the children suffered from poor absorption of their food, and 10% had parasites that further compromised their nutritional status. About 80% had what is called "leaky gut," a condition whereby the intestinal wall is too permeable, allowing foreign proteins and toxins to pass easily into the bloodstream. Almost all of these young patients had low neurotransmitter levels in their blood platelets, but their urine samples were loaded with neurotransmitters—about ten times the normal level. It appeared that many of these children had "renal leak" syndromes. That is, they were losing neurotransmitters into their urine, but these were all secondary to something that was profoundly damaging their bodies.

Every one of these children had an overly activated immune system. They all had food allergies as well as abnormally low levels of T-lymphocytes. Again, however, the basic question is: Why is this the case? The answer seems to lie, in part, with liver detoxication, something I have continued to study in detail in the context of the toxicological profile for each child.

The Liver Link Emerges

My original research dealt not only with immunological and toxicological parameters, but also with nutritional biochemistry, the gastrointestinal system, neurotransmitter levels, and perhaps most importantly, the body's detoxication systems. In 1995, after reviewing the records of my first thirty autistic patients, I presented some preliminary data in Chicago indicating that over 90 percent of the patients with autistic spectrum disorders suffer from central nervous system toxicity (neurotoxicity) caused by environmental chemicals.

These early investigations led me to believe that autism was a multifactorial disorder, a disease of many causes. One of those causes involved a breakdown in the functioning of the body's biochemical mastermind, that massive purplish organ positioned under your ribcage, the liver. The liver provides us with the right amounts of nutrients and energy to keep our lives going. It is also an essential detoxifying organ. When it functions below par, all variety of biochemical mishaps can occur. One of these is the failure to remove toxic materials that can have a highly adverse impact on brain function.

Strange as it sounds, the brain and liver share an intimate relationship. The greater the accumulation of metabolic toxins in the body, the more likely the brain will be adversely affected. In fact, there is strong evidence that problems with liver detoxication mechanisms can lead to a decline in cognitive capacities as well as a worsening of emotional health.[2] Problems related to liver detoxication are associated with a host of psychiatric illnesses and psychological problems such as chronic anxiety and irritability.[3] Under the right nutritional conditions, the two phases of liver detoxication will be balanced, and signs of neurological dysfunction and mental illness will be reduced.[4]

The most intriguing observation we drew from this first group of patients was that all of them showed certain abnormalities in liver functioning—or more specifically, in the liver's ability to detoxify substances absorbed from the diet. My basic premise concerning the etiology of the autistic spectrum of disorders relates to abnormal liver detoxication. This is already well documented. One study, for example, showed that 90 percent of the autistic subjects examined exhibited a deficiency in an enzyme in the liver called phenosulfotransferase—an enzyme intimately related to detoxication processes.[5]

Without a properly functioning liver, autistic children are highly vulnerable to the vagaries of environmental pollution. Small amounts of pollutants that would ordinarily be removed from the body begin to accumulate instead. My research suggests that these pollutants then contribute to an array of problems that collectively comprise the austistic spectrum.

Our Second Study Confirms the Liver's Role

After presenting our preliminary study to physicians and researchers at a scientific conference in Chicago, we went on to study autistic children in a more in-depth and focused fashion, this time directing our attention to the liver issue. We set out to conduct a very detailed and costly study of twenty autistic children to assess their liver detoxication capacities. Our subjects consisted of fifteen males and five females, ages three to twelve, who had been formally diagnosed with autism. The tests included caffeine clearance, glutathione conjugation, sulfation, and glucuronidation, among others. These are all part of what we refer to as the Comprehensive Liver Detoxication Evaluation (CLDE).[6]

In this study we used three laboratory tests to evaluate the evidence of toxic burden and liver detoxication in these children. First, we studied their *D-glucaric acid* levels. Elevated levels of D-glucaric acid indicate that the liver is under stress, due to chemicals, drugs, alcohol, or liver disease. We also did blood analyses to look for elevated levels of *neurotoxic (xenotiotic) chemicals*. And finally, we did the CLDE to evaluate these children's livers' ability to appropriately process the toxins they encountered.

All twenty children in our study were found to have abnormal liver detoxication. Sixteen children showed evidence of levels of toxic chemicals exceeding levels considered safe for adults; and in the two children where toxic chemical levels were not found, we found elevated glucaric acid levels, which suggests xenobiotic influences on the liver detoxication process. Overall, in this study, we found that:

- 100% of these children had abnormal liver detoxication.
- 89% had abnormal glucaric acid and 89% had abnormal mercapturic acid (both of which tell us something about the burden of neurotoxic chemicals in the body).
- 95% showed abnormal toxic chemical levels.
- 100% had abnormal skin testing.
- 100% had abnormal neurotransmitter levels.

- 100% exhibited activated immune systems.
- 100% showed abnormal nutritional deficiencies.

Without explaining what the CLDE tests mean, the bottom line is that all these ratios were imbalanced, and thus liver detoxication as a whole showed a wide range of abnormalities. The liver, as you may know, carries out the detoxication of chemical compounds in two basic phases. In phase I, chemical compounds are converted to either more or less potent compounds than the parent compounds. This renders the chemicals ready for the next stage of processing. In phase II, the so-called "conjugation phase," the toxic metabolites produced in phase I are combined (conjugated) with various molecules to make the compounds less toxic and more readily excreted.

Fiber from grains and vegetables, as well as specific nutrients such as calcium, can serve to reduce the absorption of toxic chemicals and heavy metals within the digestive tract. Additionally, a number of nutrients are needed to support each of these phases of metabolism, and this must be done in a balanced way. In particular, if phase I operates in an accelerated or exaggerated fashion, an excess of harmful metabolites will be produced, and the liver then becomes a source of toxins rather than a vehicle for getting rid of toxins. This state of "pathological detoxication" is not uncommon among autistic children, as our study showed. This is a genetic problem that can be exacerbated by high-fat foods, pesticides, drugs, alcohol, and other toxic substances. Another reason for an increased phase I level besides the genetic defect is an overabundance of toxic chemicals being processed.

Every one of the twenty autistic children in our study showed aberrant liver characteristics, and most (68%) were classified as pathological detoxifiers, while the remaining children (32%) all showed less extreme imbalances in detoxication. For the group as a whole, phase I was overly strong, while phase II was weak. This imbalance between the two phases results in huge increases in the liver's free radical production, as well as in the backup of toxins in the system. A marker for such liver-related toxicity is D-glucaric acid, and we found this to be quite high in our group of autistic children. In addition, the cysteine sulfation ratios were very high, reflecting a defect in producing sulfate (hence a weakening of phase II detoxication).

The liver's biochemical balancing act requires careful nutritional support. In particular, the phase II system must be stimulated to keep pace with the production of toxic compounds from phase I. Phase II–inducing nutrients include the phenolic antioxidants, coumarins, dithiolethiones, and thiocarbamates; these are primarily concentrated in vegetables.[7] In a recent study, extracts of common organically grown vegetables were found to contain numerous inducers of phase II detoxication systems. The richest sources were the crucifers (genus *Brassica*), which include broccoli, collards, kale, cabbages, Brussels sprouts, and many other species.[8] Other potent phase II inducers include the East Indian spice turmeric (active compound: curcumin) and N-acetyl cysteine, a precursor to the molecule glutathione. The glutathione system represents the most important detoxifying compound for all our body cells.

We also measured the blood levels of toxic chemicals found in these autistic children over an eight-month period. The list of toxins measured included benzene, xylene, styrene, chlorinated pesticides (like chloradane), PCBs, the aliphatic hydrocarbons, the hexanes, methylpentane, and others. All of these were at abnormally high levels, even compared to adults. Children are not supposed to have any toxic chemicals in their bodies. As an adult, you may accumulate some over your lifetime; however, when you find them in children, they represent a substantially greater risk, because the immune and nervous systems are more vulnerable in early life.

On a related note, I wish to emphasize that the blood is not where these harmful chemicals are usually found. Your blood provides only a superficial indicator of the true burden of these chemicals. The reason is that these chemical compounds are lipophilic (fat-loving), so they tend to concentrate in fatty tissues throughout the body. There is typically as much as a hundredfold difference between the blood and fat levels of lipophilic compounds. Thus, even when you see a seemingly small amount in the blood, it can be very meaningful from the biomedical perspective.

In this second study, published in a 1998 issue of *Toxicology and Industrial Health,* we found that 100 percent of the participants had abnormal liver detoxication and 95 percent had abnormal blood levels of toxic chemicals—levels so high that they were in excess of adult maximum ranges for good health.[9] Because body tissue is known to harbor as much as 100 times more toxic material than blood, we must assume that the true concentration of poisons in these children's brain tissue was much higher.

Our findings here only can lead to one conclusion: Autistic children have an inability to adequately detoxify a polluted environment. Again, all of the children in our group showed this basic inability to varying degrees. The Centers for Disease Control in Atlanta made note of this second study, and alerted other scientists to the possible link between environmental poisons in the body and serious nerve and tissue damage, leading to behavioral disorders and learning disabilities.

Our Third Study Unveils a Profile of Toxicity

Based on these results, we went on to conduct a *longitudinal* study of fifty-six patients who had been diagnosed with an autistic spectrum disorder, ranging in age from three to twelve. We focused our investigation on the liver detoxication profile—or how well the liver was handling toxins—and on measurements of blood levels of toxic chemicals in these children.

We found that, as in the earlier study, 54 of 55 patients whose livers we assessed had a substantial degree of abnormal liver detoxication. Only one tested within normal limits. All of these patients' livers were working out of balance. In all of them, either phase I (transforming toxic substances into more or less potent substances for processing) or phase II ("conjugation" of these substances into larger molecules that can be easily excreted) were not working properly—that is, the two phases were out of sync. This created a situation in which toxic substances that should have been neutralized and excreted from the body were instead circulating in the body in a toxic form, inflicting major damage on the brain and organ systems of the body.

In most of the children in this study—53 of the 56, or 94.6%—we also found specific neurotoxic chemicals in the bloodstream, at levels considered highly unsafe even for adults. As I mentioned earlier, toxic chemicals usually "live" in the fatty tissues of the body, not in the bloodstream—so blood levels are usually just a fraction of the actual toxic burden present in the body. Blood levels of these toxins are thought to be in a ratio of 1 to 100 with tissue levels.

It seemed obvious that an overwhelming number of autistic patients had impaired liver detoxication processes and that their bodies were under toxic chemical and heavy metal stress. We found that 98% had abnormally functioning livers and 95% had one or more toxic chemicals in their blood at levels so high they exceeded *adult* maximum ranges for good health.

Neurotoxic chemicals are found at levels many, many times what is considered to be a safe adult level, and these results are in children. These toxins are both directly and indirectly responsible for the damage to multiple organ systems, including the brain, immune system, gastrointestinal tract, pancreas, kidneys, and others.

As I mentioned earlier, most of the children in these studies also had allergies or sensitivities to foods, chemicals, and inhalants, and a defective digestive system, including malabsorption and an overgrowth of *Candida* yeast in their gastrointestinal tracts. In part because of these digestive problems, most suffered from multiple nutrient deficiencies.

Thus, in all three studies, I observed a relationship between having autism and being exposed to toxic substances. Although these studies may be criticized for their small size, autism occurs in 1 to 3 out of every 1,000 children, and thus getting enough subjects to participate can be a real challenge. More importantly, though, the testing procedures were precise and rigorously carried out. It is now up to other medical scientists to respond, and several reputable research institutions have already done so.

I clearly saw the pattern that was emerging. Autistic kids were fighting an uphill battle biologically. Their brains were being subjected to a barrage of environmental toxins. Without the right kinds of support, I reasoned, these kids were doomed to a life of extreme dysfunction.

Our Fourth Study Expands the Web of Connections

Over the past two years at my Atlanta-based center, my coworkers and I have conducted a fourth study to measure our autistic patients' improvement during various stages of treatment. Our study focused on a complex array of characteristics that make up the biological profile of autistic children. We also monitored behavioral progress using the ATEC form, which I describe in Chapter 7. We then reevaluated the patients at six-month intervals for approximately two years.

A major focus of this fourth study was the evaluation of autoimmune problems in autistic children. With the help of researchers at the Department of Neurology at Washington University in St. Louis and Immunoscience Laboratory in Beverly Hills, CA, we measured various autoantibodies—that is, antibodies generated in reaction to certain tissues within the body. These included the following: (1) antibodies to the endothelial lining of the capillaries of the temporal lobes of the brain; (2) antibodies to various components of myelin (the protective sheath surrounding nerves); (3) antibodies to oligodendrocyte, the cell that produces myelin; (4) antibodies to the glutamate (glutamic acid) receptor, which plays a vital role in various aspects of brain function; (5) antibodies to cerebellar; (6) antibodies to neuronal; and (7) antibodies to glial fibrillary acid protein. (All except the first autoantibody test were carried out by ImmunoSciences, Inc., courtesy of biochemist Arijo Vojdani, Ph.D.)

We found that approximately 51% of the children in this group had one or more of these antibodies to "self" present in their bodies. These antibodies point to a common finding in autistic children: immune dysfunction. In this particular instance, the immune system is actually attacking the tissues of the nervous system. In 1999, pediatric neurologists from Johns Hopkins Hospital reported a high correlation between autism and autoimmune disorders; they concluded that immune dysfunction could interact with various environmental factors to play a role in the development and progression of autism.[10] Animal research, if it can be extrapolated to humans, supports the possible connection between autoimmune problems and the behavioral chaos we call autism.[11] (I return to the autoimmune connection in Chapter 5, "Understanding the Autism Complex.")

What kinds of environmental factors might interact with the immune system to wreak such biological havoc? Toxic metals such as mercury, lead, and tin are one possibility. When heavy metals inflict harm on certain structures of the brain, the immune system perceives those damaged tissues as foreign, and proceeds to attack them. This process leads to a further exacerbation of the damage to the brain and other parts of the nervous system.

In our own study, my colleagues and I found that heavy metals were indeed abnormally high in these children. Specifically, about five out of every ten children had higher than normal levels of mercury, eight of every ten children had had higher than normal levels of lead, and nine of every ten had higher than normal levels of tin. Lead, mercury, and nickel are dysregulators of the immune system, and mercury, lead, and tin are neurotoxic. It is very possible that these metals were interacting with the immune system to bring about the autoimmune problems I listed above.

We were also interested in the balance of various minerals that have a beneficial impact on mental health (see Figure 1-1). Zinc was the most prevalent deficiency, followed by potassium, magnesium, and molybdenum. Of these minerals, zinc has been the most extensively studied. We found zinc deficits in six out of every ten children studied. Zinc deficiencies show a consistent link with learning and behavioral disorders, including dyslexia,[12] poor attention span,[13] and hyperactive behaviors.[14,15] Zinc is among several minerals showing the strongest correlation with autism in comparisons of hair analyses between autistic and normal children.[16] If a pregnant (or lactating) woman is low in zinc, the fetal (or infant) brain may develop incorrectly; some research suggests that this may lead to

Figure 1-1: Biochemical Findings for the Fourth Study*

Assessments of Mineral Balance in Autistic Children

Focus of Test: Minerals	Number of patients	Percent showing mineral deficiency
Zinc	72	59%
Potassium	72	45%
Magnesium	72	18%
Molybdenum	72	12%

Assessments of Heavy Metal Burden in Autistic Children

Focus of Test: Heavy Metals	Number of patients	Percent showing heavy metal excess
Tin	97	88%
Lead	97	84%
Mercury	97	51%

Assessments of Amino Acid (AA) Metabolism

Focus of Test: AA Metabolism and Digestion	Number of patients	Percent showing digestive problem or sarcosine excess
Maldigestion	85	54%
Malabsorption	85	18%
Sarcosine (indicator of chemical toxicity)	85	29%

* 51% of the children (n=73) had autoimmunity to brain tissue.

autism.[17,18,19] Note that various metal pollutants such as copper, lead, and cadmium can further deplete the body's zinc supply.

Some researchers may criticize our study for not having a control group. This is a valid criticism, of course, as the more rigorous study designs always include a control group. Our study must be considered "exploratory," designed to highlight *potential* problem areas in autistic children. Nevertheless, I believe the laboratory reference ranges used in our study provide a suitable basis for evaluating the experimental outcomes. What's clear from this study is that most (perhaps all) of these autistic children were suffering from one or more of the following: heavy metal pollution, mineral deficiencies, digestive problems, and autoimmune disorders. With just over half of the children showing some form of autoimmune reaction to brain tissues, it seems clear that the immune system plays an integral role in the development of autism.

The take-home lesson from this study is that the biological profile of autism is complex, extending beyond brain dysfunction. Autism is both *multifactorial,* involving many causes, and *systemic,* involving many parts of the body, not simply the brain. Different toxic factors affect different tissues, as some tissues are more sensitive than others. In the Appendix, you will find two flow charts, "Theoretical Mechanisms of Neurotoxicity in the Autistic Spectrum Disorders" and "Autism: A Genetic Immuno-toxicological Syndrome." These diagrams provide a visual outline and summary of the key connections I discuss in this and subsequent chapters. Such complex connections must be kept in mind when attempting to unveil the pathogenesis of autism. Clearly scientists and laypeople alike should guard against the tendency to embrace a tunnel vision perspective on this complex disorder.

A Breakthrough Perspective

At the Edelson Center for Environmental and Preventive Medicine, we have a high degree of success in treating young children who have been diagnosed as autistic. The average *rate of improvement* on our program of detoxification and nutritional support is approximately 65 percent over a two-year period.

Our approach to treating autism works because we don't focus on treating symptoms, but instead go straight to the underlying cause of the disease. Most treatments of autism even today are palliative, helping to assuage behavioral and physiological symptoms of the disorder—working to correct the problems from the outside inward. We approach the treatment of autism from just the opposite perspective, working to correct imbalances from the inside, so that improvements in behavioral symptoms follow.

It is clear to me that without understanding the underlying cause of a disease, you can't get very far in treating it. Once you know the cause, you can deal with the root of the problem. This makes for a more complete recovery. Using this approach, we have been able to reverse or substantially improve autistic symptoms in many of the autistic children I have treated.

With each child, we start by identifying the underlying cause of autism—the presence of neurotoxins in the body, and the nature of the heavy metal and toxic chemical insult to the immune and nervous systems. While we advise parents to keep their children involved with any behavioral modification therapy programs they may have begun, we focus rather on the underlying physiological mechanisms of the disease. In my experience, this is the fastest, most efficient way to attain improved functioning in these children. If you can do only one kind of treatment, this makes far more sense than one that treats only external symptoms.

The earlier autism is diagnosed, the more effective the treatment is likely to be. The longer the wait, the greater the possibility of not being able to reverse the process that is damaging the nervous system. There is too much at stake and almost no "downside"—with the exception of *certain basic side effects of therapy*—to exploring and elucidating the pathology. Our treatments related to the environmental and immunological aspects of autism are not going to cause any harm.

At the Center, when we evaluate an autistic child for treatment, we don't just look at the symptoms—we look at many facets of the person that may be playing a role in the complexity of this disorder. We study the historical, immunological, toxicological, biochemical, gastrointestinal, liver detoxication, and oxidant stress characteristics of the person. By being comprehensive, we can put together the complex picture of the origins and triggers of the illness. Without this range of information, a major piece of the "puzzle" may go unnoticed.

When parents come to me with their autistic child, the first thing I do is ask them to fill out a set of historical questionnaires that deal with the life of the child from conception to the present, as well as the life of the mother and father from the time prior to conception. We look at the potential environmental influences that may have contributed to this disease—parents' work experience, use of chemical products in the home, hobbies, dental history, and other factors—looking for any and all clues. We also ask for details of the child's birth, medical history, nutritional profile, allergies, and symptoms of autism.

The child is then given a thorough physical examination. Laboratory evaluations to be performed include blood, urine, and stool tests. These tests are quite specialized and yield information about the origin of the illness and the reasons for some of the symptoms associated with the illness.

The tests we perform on each child include: immunological, intradermal skin or blood testing for allergies, heavy metal toxicity panel, digestive characteristics, gastrointestinal evaluation, free radical investigation, nutritional evaluation, liver detoxication profile, and toxic chemical blood levels.

This is an extensive evaluation, but it is all very important in putting together the puzzle pieces so that we can explain the illness completely. By dealing with only one aspect of the illness, we might be able to improve the child's level of functioning to some degree, but we want to know all of the immunological and biochemical problems or factors, so that we can achieve the most productive course of healing.

Once the evaluation process is complete, the next step is to design a comprehensive therapeutic plan. Plans vary to meet the needs of each patient. They may include any or all of the following treatments:

- Nutritional supplementation
- Immunotherapy (if allergies are present)
- Environmental controls
- Removal of chemicals and metals
- Intravenous gamma globulin (if indicated)
- Anticandida therapy (if needed)
- Healing of the gastrointestinal tract
- Maldigestion correction
- Liver detoxication upregulation

We also strongly recommend that any behavioral and educational techniques being used to improve day-to-day functioning be continued, and be considered part of this multidimensional therapeutic plan.

We hope that by bringing some much-needed "light" to this subject we can finally begin to show the parents of autistic children that they do not have to be satisfied with only slight improvements. They can "shoot for the moon"—attempt to help their children attain greatly improved behavior and cerebral function. With our thorough and comprehensive approach, I believe that it is possible in certain cases to reverse this disease completely, and in others to make major improvements.

My research in clinical molecular medicine indicates that autistic people are trapped in a biochemical quagmire rooted in a genetic flaw in the body's ability to neutralize and eliminate harmful chemicals and metals. I believe the disease originates in fetal exposure to environmental pollution during pregnancy. We need to keep in mind, however, that the mother's toxic burden prior to pregnancy is shifted to the fetus during pregnancy. After birth, the infant is incapable of adequately neutralizing a wide range of chemical and metal pollutants, resulting in undue toxicity to the brain. Normally such chemicals would not so dramatically threaten our physical and mental health. For individuals predisposed to autism, however, such a toxic burden can have tragic and long-lasting consequences.

Thankfully, we can attack the roots of this disease once it has developed. Our genetic makeup provides only the basic plan or blueprint upon which life unfolds. It is up to us to provide the building materials, which come from our food and water supply. We are architects and builders both. Best of all, the building itself—our body's intricate design—can be renovated. And *that* is the exciting task of specialists in environmental medicine as well as in the emerging field of clinical molecular medicine (the type of medicine I practice, which includes applied immunology, applied toxicology, free radical biology, and nutritional biochemistry).

Matthew's Story

Now I would like to share with you the story of one of my young patients who benefited remarkably from our unique approach to treating this disease.

When I first met Matthew Colburn a little more than a year ago, he sat quietly in a chair in my office, making no eye contact with anyone, including his mother. He didn't say a word. When Matthew's mother Theresa brought him to see me in June 1999, three-year-old Matthew had recently been diagnosed with severe autism. He seemed removed from everything around him, lost in a tunnel of silence that no one could penetrate, much less understand.

Like many autistic children, Matthew had appeared normal for the first year of his life. He grew like other babies, crawled like others, and started

walking soon after his first birthday. At fifteen months he seemed excep-
tionally quiet—at least compared to other children his age—but not quiet
enough to cause alarm. At age two, Matthew was still not talking, although
he ran about the house and played with his toys. This, too, didn't seem abnormal since not all two-year-olds talk. Matthew could have had what pediatricians call a developmental delay. The family doctor assured Theresa
that her son was probably just a "slow grower."

But there were certain perplexing signs as well, such as Matthew's
habit of spinning wheels on a stroller, walking on his toes, and running in
repeated circles around the table. He also had an obsession with opening
and closing drawers and doors repeatedly for long periods of time. Several
months after Matthew's second birthday, Theresa's mother Jane sat next to
a two-year-old boy during a cross-country flight. She noticed a startling
difference between the child and her grandson. "He laughed and talked
and made regular eye contact with me," Jane told Theresa. She urged her
daughter to take Matthew to local child development experts.

Theresa, who is a single mom (she's divorced), thought about it and
then agreed. The following month, in August 1999, Matthew was evaluated by a team of specialists—a developmental pediatrician, an occupational therapist, a speech therapist, a neurologist, and a child psychologist.
Their diagnosis struck Theresa with devastating force: severe autism.
They recommended speech and language therapy and behavioral modification.

"They told me he would probably end up in an institution," Theresa told
me with a shudder. "They said he was not just autistic, but highly autistic,
that he would always have problems with expressing himself." She said she
had read that many severely autistic children never go beyond babbling or
making bizarre sounds, and she feared that her son would grow up feeling
tormented by his inability to interact normally with others.

"Dr. Edelson, I'm not ready to accept that," Theresa concluded. "There
has to be a way to reach Matthew."

At that time, Matthew was as quiet and removed as a Zen monk. He
would fixate on certain objects for long periods of time. He preferred to
play alone, and his favorite toy was a wooden block bear, a four-piece peg
puzzle he carried around and was obsessively attached to. If the toy was
misplaced or moved, Matthew would simply "flip out," to use Theresa's
phrase. He'd begin to utter long piercing shrieks that made Theresa and
her daughter want to cover their ears.

Like other autistic children, Matthew seemed most content when everything followed a highly predictable routine. When Theresa took him out in the carriage for one of her regular runs, he insisted on maintaining the same route every time. If she turned down a different path, or even if she tried to run a bit farther than usual, he threw a tantrum. The same fetish for routine applied to his clothes. He loved a certain pair of sandals and wore them everywhere. When Theresa bought him new shoes, he screamed until he had his sandals back.

Everything in Matthew's profile pointed to a syndrome that I recognized. After hearing Theresa's story, I proposed that we do a battery of tests to determine Matthew's levels of chemical toxins and heavy metals, as well as his liver and immune function. I told Theresa I thought we could help her son.

"We're not going to focus on his autistic behavior," I cautioned. "We need to focus on what's going on with Matthew internally, on the biological forces that could be driving this behavior." Theresa nodded. Her own research had led her to the same point. We had to unravel the cause of this disease, not just treat its symptoms.

The following week, Theresa and Matthew began commuting to our clinic in Atlanta for testing. The core of our program is detoxification—using supplements and therapies to help correct defective liver functioning and to accelerate the body's own ability to eliminate poisons. We began by running a series of tests on Matthew to determine the levels of toxins in his blood, hair, and urine, how well his immune and digestive systems were functioning, and whether he had allergies or sensitivities.

Sure enough, Matthew's test results revealed that the levels of certain key chemicals were much higher than normal: hexane, 40 times higher; 3-methyl pentane, 10 times higher; styrene, 2 times higher; and 2-methyl pentane, 5 times higher. On top of this, he had a classic malabsorption syndrome, which meant that he could not absorb a wide variety of nutrients. He also had an overgrowth of yeast in his intestines and a host of allergies to foods, dyes, inhalants, and preservatives. And his hair and red blood cells showed moderately high lead levels.

Matthew's test results came as no surprise. The liver function tests alone gave me a lot of information about the toxic burden in Matthew's body. Lab tests showed that Matthew's liver, as the primary detoxication organ, was markedly impaired in its ability to flush toxins out of his body. Matthew had a biochemical profile that was classically autistic. Had we not found those high levels of toxins, I would have been shocked.

What followed was seven weeks of day-long treatments (four consecutive weeks, two off, and then three more consecutive weeks) designed to alleviate the toxic burden. These included exercise, sauna, massage, and numerous supplements (high-dose multivitamins, glycine, glutathione, glutamine, magnesium, calcium, zinc, acetyl-L-carnitine, and cilantro) designed to strengthen the liver, as well as the digestive, immune, and nervous systems. Matthew was also taken off wheat and dairy—a real challenge for Theresa, who also had to monitor for dyes and preservatives in Matthew's foods.

Much to Theresa's amazement, Matthew tolerated the supplements well. The sauna, however, was another story. Because the skin is the body's largest organ. and sweat carries with it toxins from the bloodstream, the sauna plays an important role in this process. To make it easier for Matthew, Theresa did this portion of the treatments with him. Before entering the sauna, Theresa and Matthew were supposed to walk on a treadmill for ten minutes to increase their blood circulation. Theresa reported that Matthew would last about five minutes before he started to cheat, putting one foot down on the side and just working one leg at a time. Some days he'd last only seven minutes before becoming bored.

Then it was time to enter the sauna, in which temperatures ranged from 140 to 160 degrees Fahrenheit. The two of them were supposed to sit in the sauna for thirty minutes, and Theresa was supposed to wipe the sweat from Matthew constantly so that his body would not reabsorb the toxins. But the first time inside, Matthew began pitching a fit within five minutes, and five minutes later Theresa had to pull him out.

A television installed just outside the sauna—and visible from inside—solved the problem. Watching videos of the children's show *Barney* helped to calm Matthew. By the end of the week, Matthew's body had adjusted, and he began to relax into the sauna experience. Eventually he was able to stay for fifteen, twenty, and finally thirty minutes.

The sauna was followed by a shower and then a massage of the fatty tissues to help coax yet more toxins out through the lymphatic system. The cycle was repeated four times a day for a week at a time. And each day Matthew drank two quarts of water—spiked with a little white grape juice to make it more palatable—to help flush the waste products from his body.

A few weeks into Matthew's treatment, the first changes became noticeable. Matthew was more attentive and alert. But the biggest change came during week four when Matthew started to say his first words, "juice" and "mommy."

"[From that point] every new word made me feel elated to the point of crying," says Theresa. "I could see he was beginning to get it, but then I could never be sure if he would remember it the next time. Then one morning we came back from the Edelson Center and he said 'bagel' when he wanted one. At that point, I could see he was choosing his words. It's so profoundly moving. It feels like a great mystery is unfolding with each breakthrough."

About half of all autistic children never speak. And those that do speak often use language in unusual ways and aren't capable of associating words with actual objects. But after six weeks, Matthew had shown a 30 percent improvement based on speech-language tests. After seven weeks of treatment, all four chemical toxins had dropped to within normal limits.

In the months that followed, Theresa tried more conventional autism treatments, like auditory integration training for his overly sensitive hearing and occupational therapy to improve his motor skills. Matthew also benefited from the Lovaas method of behavior modification, a set of techniques that help autistic children learn, become more socially acceptable, and reduce compulsive behaviors that interfere with their ability to learn new skills. I have no doubt that all these therapies worked together with our detoxification program to account for Matthew's dramatic recovery.

Today, at four years of age, Matthew laughs, plays, and interacts with others. Gone is the lack of eye contact. Gone is the tunnel of silence. Matthew actually seems to welcome new experiences. When visitors come to the house, he will climb into their laps and look into their eyes. If Theresa wants to run a different route or buy Matthew a new pair of shoes, he's okay with the change.

In the latter half of the year 2000, Matthew's objective improvement, based on the ATEC test (see Chapter 7), was 63 percent—an indication that he had indeed made amazing progress. In terms of his gross motor skills and coordination (walking, for example), Matthew is at a normal age level. His fine motor skills (like holding a pencil) have improved tremendously and are quickly approaching normal.

Matthew's main weakness, at this point, lies in his verbal skills, which are a little more than a year behind schedule. Now and then he adds another word to his vocabulary. He cannot, however, string several long sentences together or speak in complex sentences—though he is beginning to put complex sentences together. Nevertheless, the fact that Matthew speaks as well as he does is an amazing accomplishment. "None of the behavioral therapists we're working with have seen a severely autistic child become verbal in such a short time," Theresa told me. "Also, they cannot believe that he has picked up lessons so fast and mastered them. For most autistic kids, it takes a week to just get them to stay in the chair without throwing a temper tantrum. Matthew came into the chair immediately and on his own, and he has actually shown an eagerness to learn new things."

Our most recent follow-up evaluations of Matthew, in early 2001, revealed that his body's toxic burden had been greatly reduced. Nonetheless, a substantial burden remained. In addition to ongoing problems with digestion, we identified various biochemical imbalances. These included the following: heavy losses of tryptophan via the urine (possibly due to chemical toxicity); high sarcosine levels, indicating toxicity; an increase in creatinine levels, suggesting mild kidney damage that was most likely toxin-related; low glutathione levels, probably due to excessive oxidative stress; and low but still worrisome levels of lead, and high levels of two other heavy metals, arsenic and antimony. Matthew continued to show some abnormalities in his liver functioning, specifically an inability to flush out toxins (phase II). These persistent problems suggest that Matthew would benefit from chelation, modulation of liver functions, and other specialized detoxification strategies.

Matthew still takes his supplements, and he invites his mother to take saunas with him. They have installed one in their home (along with a TV), something I encourage all my patients to do if they can afford it. During the sauna, Matthew checks the temperature with his mother to make sure it's correct. He says, "Check temperature, check temperature." When the beeper goes off to indicate the end of 30 minutes, Matthew says, "All done with sauna."

It is hard not to ascribe a major part of Matthew's rapid improvement to the detoxification strategies that make up the backbone of my therapeutic approach. "Matthew is no longer tuned out and he has learned language and new skills much faster than any of the Lovaas or OT specialists expected," says Theresa. "I don't believe he would have done nearly as well without having first gone through the program in Atlanta. Without the detox work, I doubt he'd be anywhere near where he is now."

There is little doubt that Matthew has benefited tremendously from all the behavioral modification and speech therapy work as well. Many autistic children learn to control their behavior through these techniques alone, but they never completely transform the internal conditions that drive the aberrant behavior in the first place. I am now convinced, based on my observations of these children over the past five years, that you can do all the

Lovaas in the world, but if you don't focus on the biological level first, you simply won't get rapid or long-lasting results. The consequence of using such behavior modification techniques alone, without addressing the underlying biological problem, is that the child's behavior becomes more controllable and predictable. The end result, however, is a child who responds in a robotic fashion to cues from the parents—not a child who thinks and acts with some measure of fluidity and autonomy.

When Theresa looks back, she can't believe how far they've come. "My parents told me the other day that the biggest change of all is that Matthew is a happy child now," she told me recently. "This means the world to me. All the blood and sweat, all the hard work, has paid off. He's a totally different boy now. He speaks, which is a miracle in itself. He's even naughty at times, and I love it. He'll look me in the eye when he's getting into mischief. I know the healing work isn't over yet, but I'm very optimistic that he's going to be okay."

Keys to Successful Therapy

After treating and observing more than 200 autistic children, it has become clear to me that these children have certain environmental risk factors in common. These common denominators constitute a kind of profile of environmental stress. Here's the basic profile:

1. All suffered from toxic chemical and heavy metal burdens, and most also showed drastic nutritional deficiencies.
2. All showed allergies or abnormal sensitivities toward their environment—toward foods, chemicals, and inhalants—though in most cases these sensitivities were hidden. There is now incontrovertible evidence of injury to the immune system.
3. All showed evidence of abnormal functioning of the liver, the body's key organ for detoxication. This probably arises from a convergence of genetic, nutritional, and environmental factors.

My experience with these children has led me to investigate more deeply the roots of environmental illnesses. Those studies, combined with my personal experience, have reinforced my growing conviction that autism is the result of both faulty genes and a polluted environment. I am certain that this unfortunate combination plays a profoundly important role in other childhood behavioral disorders as well—a massive epidemic that is sweeping not only the United States, but most of the industrialized world.

The key to successful therapy, then, depends on how we deal with the toxic burden these children face. My program is aimed at removing the burden as rapidly as possible. Parents of the children I treat tell me that over the course of approximately two years—a typical time frame for treatment—their children more than double their ability to learn and communicate more effectively with others. Formerly autistic children approach normal function.

But this represents only a handful of all the autistic children. What about the thousands, perhaps millions, of others whose parents know only that their child is unhappy, uncommunicative, unloving—or at the other extreme, hyperactive, excitable, anxious, and unable to concentrate—and do not know why or what to do about it?

To date, my track record with this multifaceted approach to autism is strong, and I hope to strengthen it further in the coming years with more rigorous studies of larger groups of children. I'm constantly—some might say obsessively—striving to learn more about, and do more for these children. As I tell other physicians working in this field, I am entirely open to examining new approaches to treatment that will give children with autism and learning disabilities a better chance at life. It is this strong desire to help children recover from the tragic reality of mindblindness that has prompted me to write this book.

Figure 1-2

A Summary of My Research in Environmental Medicine

Based on the research I've presented in this chapter, I consider the most common causes to be: (1) molecular damage from environmental factors, caused by toxic chemicals and heavy metals; (2) an aberrantly functioning liver detoxication system; (3) environmental hypersensitivity caused by an injured immune system; (4) biochemical imbalances resulting from numerous factors, including maldigestion, malabsorption, and rapid depletion of nutrients used to deal with the toxic burden; (5) poor dietary habits, resulting in nutritional imbalances that reinforce these other problems; (6) autoimmune pathology causing the symptoms and signs found in the autistic spectrum; and (7) a possibility that a genetic defect exists in the metallothionein protein formation.

Chapter 2

◆

As Through a
Clouded Window

Monica, a three-year-old girl with wispy dark blond hair and deep-set eyes, is sitting on the living room floor. She plays silently with her favorite stuffed animal, a small white dog. She is dressed neatly in a blue-and-green-plaid dress with a white collar.

Monica plays intently, petting the top of the little dog's head, not looking up when her father calls to her, "Come here, Monica!" She studies the dog with a look of intense concentration, seemingly unaware of her father's voice. "Monica!" He tries again but there is no response. He comes over, kneels on the floor next to her, gently lifts her up, and puts her into a small chair. Immediately she begins moaning as though in pain, fighting off his arms, arching her back as her voice rises to a shriek of terror. "Good job!" her father says gently as he holds her in the chair.

Born in January 1991, Monica at first gave every appearance of being a normal child. She was cheerful and loved to be around people. Like parents everywhere, Monica's parents were thrilled when she learned to crawl, teethe, walk, and speak her first words. But when Monica was two and a half, an ominous change began to take place. She stopped learning new words, and then she stopped using many of the words she had once known.

Around that time, in June 1993, Monica was diagnosed with classic autism. She and her parents began a program of behavioral modification therapy. By the age of three, Monica had stopped speaking entirely. When I spoke with her parents soon afterward, they were understandably bewildered and heartbroken.

Monica did find ways to communicate, but only through glances and hand gestures. More often, she did not ask but merely stood still and waited for her parents to figure out what she needed or wanted—for instance, a drink of water or a toy. She began to withdraw from the world, no longer answering when her parents called her, her face no longer lighting up the way it once had. She shrank from any human touch. When her parents picked her up, she screamed and fought. She kept her stuffed animals lined up neatly in a row on her windowsill, and would scream and sob if she ever found one that was not in the place where she had left it. It was as though the person Monica had been had been spirited away, and replaced by this somber and fearful little being.

I know that Monica's story is an all-too-familiar scenario for parents of autistic children. A number of the parents I've interviewed say they feel as though they have inexplicably lost their child to a dark and sinister force, or perhaps to a hostile, fearful stranger. As one father put it, "It is as though my son had died to his previous existence, and begun a new one as a stranger." There is growing evidence that autism begins during fetal development; even so, full-blown autistic symptoms may not appear until much later. Classic autism usually manifests itself between the ages of eighteen and thirty-six months. In the earliest stages of the disease, it is often difficult to tell the difference between normal behavioral idiosyncrasies and autistic symptoms.

Throughout this book, I will be describing or alluding to what I consider to be the most salient biological mechanisms behind autism. Nonetheless, many of the mechanisms that drive this disorder have yet to be mapped out. Autism is still recognized and diagnosed almost exclusively through its behavioral symptoms. In young children the signs of the disorder are puzzling but distinctly recognizable—behavior such as rocking, recoiling from being touched or held, becoming fixated on a particular object, toe walking, hand flapping, tantrums, an obsessive desire for sameness, and a fear of even the smallest change in the environment. Autism has been aptly called "mindblindness" because it is also characterized by a deficiency in perceiving the subtleties of social interactions, or "reading the minds" of other people for social cues. For the person with an autistic spectrum disorder, social interactions are never easy, and may require mastering a set of skills that don't come naturally.

Three out of four people diagnosed with autism are also diagnosed with some degree of mental retardation. And an estimated one third of autistic children also suffer from seizures. About one in ten autistic people displays exceptional abilities in skills such as art or memorization of numbers or names. Perhaps one in a hundred are identified as savants because of their remarkable abilities. Intriguingly, if a child begins to recover from the debilitating symptoms of autism through treatment, these exceptional abilities seem to disappear along with the illness.

A diagnosis of autism can be the beginning of a long struggle for a child's parents, who must watch their son or daughter retreat into a mysterious and lonely world they cannot enter. They must endure daily tantrums, obsessive behavior, special education programs, endless trips to doctors and behavioral therapists. The outcome of these therapeutic efforts is never guaranteed. In severe cases, autistic children may never be able to function on their own, while those with milder cases of autism may go on to have independent and productive lives as adults.

Though the disease was once regarded as a psychiatric disorder, it is now clear that autism is a neurological disorder. For reasons we do not yet understand, 80% or four out of every five autistic children are male. The range of symptoms of autism and autism-like conditions—known as autism spectrum disorders or the pervasive developmental disorders (PDD)—is even more varied than the labels that we have tried to develop to classify them. In addition to classical autism, the autistic spectrum includes an array of aberrant behavioral disorders, as I'll discuss shortly.

The theories of the cause of autism are also diverse. Is autism genetic? Environmental? Caused by some dysfunction in the home? For decades, most psychiatrists viewed autism as a psychological disorder, caused by poor parenting. We now know that autism is caused by biological factors, but there is little agreement over which specific factors are most critical, and exactly how they cause autism.

Researchers agree that genetic predisposition has something to do with it, since autism seems to run in families. This does not mean, however, that autism is transferred in a neat and predictable fashion from the parents to the offspring. Instead, recent research suggests that environmental toxicity, such as lead poisoning and a preservative called thimerosal in vaccines, may play some role in triggering the disease. Indeed, as our first study showed, there is now compelling evidence for an environmental link with autism.[1] The incidence of this disorder continues to increase, and now surpasses both childhood cancer and Down syndrome.

Autism used to be relatively rare, but its incidence has risen dramatically since the late 1980s. Environmentally polluted areas have shown a clustering of autistic cases, which suggests that exposure of a developing nervous system to toxic agents may lead to neurological damage characteristic of autistic syndrome. For instance, the U.S. Centers for Disease Control have confirmed a high concentration of autistic cases in the working-class town of Brick Township, New Jersey, which also happens to harbor a large toxic landfill. I describe the rising trends and the situation at Brick Township in greater detail in Chapter 3.

Diagnosing Autism

The disorder called autism was first identified by physician Leo Kanner in 1938. Before that, from around 1800 to 1938, the disorder had been widely known as "childhood schizophrenia." In 1943, Dr. Kanner identified eleven autistic patients who exhibited impaired language skills, an obsessive desire for sameness, and "extreme autistic aloneness." These were children who seemed to be operating in a world of their mind's own creation, a world quite apart from that of healthy, nonautistic people. The word *autism* comes from the Greek root words *autos* and *isma*—literally, a condition of "self-involvement."

Even after Kanner identified it, the disorder remained relatively rare until about 1960. It was not yet recognized as a neurological disorder, but was thought to be a psychiatric disorder attributed to a range of possible causes, including genetics, mental illness, and poor parenting. We now know that autism and its associated behaviors occur in more than 1 in 500 individuals. It is conservatively estimated that nearly 400,000 people in the United States today have autism, and the rates of this illness appear to be rising rapidly, not only in the United States but worldwide. We'll take a closer look at this rising rate and its possible causes in the next chapter.

Because we have no definitive diagnostic tests for the biological manifestations of autism, it remains one of the only neurological disorders that must be diagnosed almost entirely through behavioral symptoms. To further complicate matters, autism is frequently found alongside other problems, such as mental retardation, severe language impairment, hyperactivity, attention deficit disorder (ADD), or epilepsy, which can make the disorder more difficult to recognize.

We know that autism interferes with the normal development of the brain in the areas of reasoning, social interaction, communication skills, and emotions such as love and empathy. Children and adults with autism typically have deficiencies in verbal and nonverbal communication, social interactions, and leisure or play activities. Autistic people may exhibit repeated body movements such as hand flapping, rocking, or spinning; they may have unusual responses to people or attachments to objects; and they may resist changes in routines. In some cases they may exhibit aggressive or self-injurious behavior.

Autism is characterized by a complex constellation of behaviors. Any of the following symptoms may indicate the presence of autism in a child.

- Marked lack of awareness of the existence of feelings of others
- Absence of, or abnormal seeking of, comfort at times of distress
- Absence of or impaired imitation
- Impairment in making peer relationships
- No mode of communication, such as communicative babbling, facial expression, gesture, mime, or spoken language
- Abnormal nonverbal communication, with lack of eye-to-eye gaze, facial expressions, or body posture
- Absence of imaginative activity: play-acting, adult roles, fantasy characters, lack of interest in imaginary events
- Abnormalities in speech: volume, pitch, stress, rate, rhythm, and intonation
- Impairment in ability to initiate or sustain a conversation with others despite adequate speech
- Stereotyped body movements: hand flicking, twisting, spinning, head banging, complex whole-body movements
- Persistent preoccupation with parts of objects
- Marked distress with changes in trivial aspects of environment, such as an item being moved from its usual spot
- Unreasonable insistence on following routines in precise detail
- Markedly restricted range of interests and a preoccupation with one narrow interest

According to the fourth edition of the *Diagnosis and Statistical Manual of Mental Disorders,* or DSM-IV, published by the American Psychiatric Association, autism is classified as a Pervasive Developmental Disorder (PDD) characterized by twelve diagnostic criteria. These criteria fall into three categories—impairments in social interaction, impairments in communication, and a restricted repertoire of activities and interests. A diagnosis of autism requires that a child display at least six of these twelve symptoms, with a minimum number in each category.

If a child does not fit the definition of autism given above, he or she may be diagnosed with a condition called Pervasive Developmental Disorder Not Otherwise Specified (PDD-NOS). Such a diagnosis of non-specific forms of Pervasive Developmental Disorder (PDD) may include atypical types of autism that do not fall into the above categories because of late age of onset, for example, or subthreshold or atypical symptoms. According to the DSM-IV, this diagnosis is to be used when autistic-like behaviors are present—in particular, when there is severe impairment in the development of social and verbal communication skills—but the child does not meet the criteria for classic autism or any other specific Pervasive Developmental Disorder, Schizophrenia, Schizotypal Personality Disorder, or Avoidant Personality Disorder.[2]

The Autistic Spectrum

Autism is not really a single disorder, but a continuum of conditions. These range from milder disorders such as Asperger's syndrome to debilitating forms of classic autism, in which the patient is unable to speak or walk normally. The autistic disorders as a group have been variously referred to as childhood autism, infantile autism, autistic disorder, pervasive developmental disorder (PDD), and childhood psychosis. One theory suggests that the current epidemic is not the same illness that Kanner describes in 1938, but a "new illness" with certain differences from the original description. This new process is related to toxic injury—the old one wasn't an epidemic and may have been a different disorder.

Figure 2-1

Asperger's—>	PDD-NOS—>	Autism
(less severe)	(more severe)	(most severe)

What do these "autistic spectrum" disorders have in common? Many adults who suffer from learning disabilities also exhibit symptoms of autistic syndrome. The greater the learning disability, the higher the number of autistic traits tends to be.[3] However subtle the manifestation of symptoms, all of these disorders exhibit varying degrees of the three main categories of autistic impairment—impairments in social interaction, impairments in communication, and a restricted range of activities and interests.

At the severe end of the spectrum is a more impaired group with greater developmental compromise, social aloofness, and a larger number of autistic symptoms, while at the milder end is a less impaired group with higher intelligence quotients (IQ), more socially integrated behavior, and fewer autistic symptoms.[4] While the lower-functioning group is clearly defined according to DSM-IV criteria, the higher-functioning group is less well defined, with no separate category of its own, falling instead into subcategories of autistic disorder or PDD-NOS. This may contribute to difficulty in recognizing these disorders for what they are, instead of dismissing them as simple social maladjustment or learning difficulties.

Asperger's syndrome is one such high-functioning autistic disorder. Unlike classic autism, it does not have its own DSM-IV diagnostic category. The disorder was discovered by Hans Asperger, a Viennese pediatrician, in the 1940s; his work then went unnoticed for several decades, but was rediscovered in the early 1980s. Symptoms of this disorder—as well as other autistic spectrum disorders—may include repetitive speech, monotonic voice, coordination problems, depression, dislike of change, adherence to routines and rituals, and difficulty in relating normally to other people, particularly in social situations. It is far more common in boys than in girls. Most individuals have normal or above-average IQ. Asperger's and autism should be thought of as two qualitatively similar points on a scale of severity, rather than as two separate disorders.[5] Asperger's is often not adequately diagnosed and treated, because it is not as easily recognized as classic autism. For the Asperger's sufferer, who may often feel like an awkward social outsider, finding a name for this malady in itself can be a tremendous relief.

These autistic patterns also appear to run in families. Parents or siblings of autistic people sometimes exhibit milder versions of autistic spectrum disorders. The autistic *phenotype*—that is, its outward characteristics or usual pattern of expression—includes a range of milder social and language-based cognitive impairments. Neurobiologic studies suggest that these traits have to do with abnormalities in the cerebellum, the cortex, and the limbic structures of the brain.[6] One study of parents who had two autistic children found that these parents exhibited traits milder than, but qualitatively similar to, autism. Compared to another group of parents of children with Down syndrome, these parents' personalities tended toward rigidity, aloofness, hypersensitivity to criticism, and anxiety, as well as speech and language impairments and more limited friendships than the parents in the other group.[7] (In later chapters I delve into some of the underlying causes of these problems based on my research in environmental medicine.)

In another study, the parents of two autistic children exhibited significantly greater cognitive deficits than the parents of a Down syndrome child, suggesting that a cognitive deficit may itself be, in some cases, an expression of a genetic predisposition to autism.[8] In general, relatives within families that have multiple-incidence autism tend to exhibit higher communication deficits and behaviors that are milder but qualitatively similar to autism.[9] These studies suggest that the DSM-IV-designated autistic spectrum disorders are only part of the picture—there appear to be degrees of autistic behavior that are part of the autism phenotype, but not necessarily diagnosable as disease. We may not be able to put these disorders into a box with a name on it, but all have the same abnormal biology, with different phenotypes. These phenomena may eventually give us more insight into the nature of the autistic disorder, as well as the role genetic factors play in its development.

Most of my patients with autistic spectrum disorders suffer from serious language impairments, though they may actually excel in areas of visual or spatial perception and expression. In communicating with autistic children, the use of visual cues rather than auditory language has been shown to work better in many cases.[10] Early language deficits have been correlated with other autistic symptoms, such as toe walking, lower IQ, and social impairment.[11,12] At the same time, autistic children who exhibit useful speech at age two tend to fare better in the short term than children who do not.[13] Many autistic children also suffer from oversensitivity to sound, touch, or other sensory information.

The autistic patterns expressed in this range of disorders exhibit not only certain characteristic weaknesses, but also unique strengths. Several studies have demonstrated that people suffering from autistic spectrum disorders have impaired social interaction and verbal fluency—they are less able to interpret social cues and adapt to new situations—while they seem to excel at other tasks, such as memorization. They also exhibit superior spatial perception. One theory that may help explain this is that if certain areas of the brain are hypofunctioning, others are hyperfunctioning, compensating for decreased activity in those damaged areas of the brain.

Researchers at Cambridge University recently developed a new tool for determining where a person falls on the "autistic spectrum." The test, called the Autism Quotient (AQ), scores the person on a scale of 0 to 50, with a higher score representing a higher level of autism. The researchers were particularly interested in so-called "high-functioning autism." They administered the test to four groups—58 adults with Asperger's syndrome (AS) or high-functioning autism (HFA), 840 Cambridge University students, 16 winners of the UK Mathematics Olympiad, and 174 randomly selected controls. Eighty percent of the AS/HFA group scored 32 or higher on the test, with only 2% of controls scoring this high. In general, men scored higher on the test than women. While the Cambridge students scored similarly to the control group, the science and math students scored significantly higher on the test than humanities and social science students. Researchers concluded that this test could be a valuable tool for diagnosing autism in high-functioning individuals.[14]

Mindblindness is a term that has been used to describe the inner state of people who have autistic spectrum disorders, particularly classic autism and high-functioning autistic disorders like Asperger's syndrome. This is the inability to "read" other people's minds, to pick up on social cues such as tone of voice and facial expression. The same Cambridge research group also conducted a study in which three high-functioning adults with Asperger's were asked to look at photos of pairs of eyes and identify what emotion was expressed—preoccupied, serious, grateful, imploring, and the like. The subjects were a mathematician, a physicist, and a computer scientist.

The result? They were completely at a loss in trying to decipher the emotions expressed by the eyes in the pictures. In another study, eight high-functioning children with autism and verbal IQ above 70 were tested. The children were able to infer the meanings of certain words for mental states from related verbs. However, they were unable to infer what certain verbs implied about mental states, to make inferences about social scripts, or to understand metaphor. All of these tasks would have required an understanding of social context.[15] Autistic children also have difficulties with abstract thought—they tend to process sensory information directly, without forming abstract categories through which to understand the information.

Such tendencies are reflected in the way autistic children play with each other.[16] A child with Asperger's might not understand the nuances of social banter. He may take a joke literally and think someone is trying to start a fight with him, or abruptly leave a conversation when he has finished his part in it without understanding that the other person may not be finished, or he may go on and on about some pet topic without realizing that he is boring the other person.[17] Echolalia, a symptom of autism in which the child echoes the speech of others instead of replying, may occur when a child is spoken to and senses the need for a response. If he is not sure what kind of response is required, he may simply echo the question, hoping that will suffice.

The following scenario further illustrates the phenomenon of mind-blindness. Two children are watching the following scene, an autistic child and a normal child. Lisa puts a marble in a basket, puts the lid on, and leaves the room. Her friend Bill comes in while she's gone, moves the marble into a covered box, and puts the lid back on both. Then Lisa comes back into the room. The two containers look just as they did when she left them. Which one will she look in to find the marble? A normal four-year-old will say that Lisa will look in the basket, where she left it. A four-year-old autistic child will be more likely to predict that Lisa will look in the box for the marble, since that's where it is. The autistic child, in other words, has trouble putting herself in Lisa's place, or anticipating how Lisa would experience the world.[18]

With great effort, some people with autistic disorders can learn to navigate social interactions by developing their own devices for interpreting such cues. However, many never feel comfortable in social situations. One autistic patient explains how he learned to manage the problem of eye contact.

I learned to smile and hold my face in people's direction. Even without eye contact, walking nice and maintaining my posture took a lot of thinking and concentration. I used pseudo-eye contact when someone was still far from me and would make a mild friendly generic smile as one might on a pleasant day towards a stranger walking in the park. That way if I didn't know the person it would not be too inappropriate and if I did know the person I wouldn't be ignoring them. Then I would look down as if I was concentrating on something else, or as if I were a little shy or submissive (the opposite of my true nature) but I believed it was better I looked shy than stupid.[19]

The socially inept "nerdy" scientist image may be more than a stereotype. Asperger's syndrome and other high-functioning autistic syndromes have long been associated with exceptional scientific and mathematical skills. Both classical autism and Asperger's disorders are associated with impaired movement. Asperger's has long been associated with clumsiness, while autism has been shown to be associated in some individuals with impulsive behaviors or a general lack of anticipation in motor activity.[20] Both conditions also reveal similar motor coordination impairment as it is expressed in handwriting—individuals with an autism spectrum disorder tend to exhibit macrographia, or large (and often poorly formed) handwriting.[21] The flip side of this condition is an ability to concentrate intensely, to go deeply into one subject or area of research, to be calm and attend logically to detail rather than reacting emotionally to situations. Simon Baron-Cohen of Cambridge University recounts the story of a couple who lost their child in the zoo—the mother became extremely upset, while the father, who suffered from Asperger's, was able to logically conduct a search for the child, and found him.

About one in every ten autistic people has an extraordinary talent, usually in a very narrow area. An autistic person might be able to tell you exactly what day of the week you were born on, or recite pages out of the phone book from memory. Some autistic people excel in art or poetry or musical performance. Perhaps one in every hundred is identified as a savant, a mathematical or artistic genius who possesses truly astounding abilities. This is particularly fascinating since the very talents these people exhibit are symptomatic of their disorder—they may perform tasks with remarkable skill, yet in a narrow or inflexible manner.[22] Their skills, in mathematics for example, may not always be related to IQ, but may be related to how they approach the task. On the other hand, there may also be fewer differences than expected between a normal person and one with autism. Researchers at Oxford University compared the work of a savant poet to that of a normal poet. The verbal patterns the two poets employed were similar, though the savant poet's work referred more often to self-analysis and less often to descriptions of people not related to the self. Both made ample use of simile and metaphor.[23]

Sometimes autistic children with severely limited verbal capacity will display a startling ability to draw natural scenes from memory, with astonishing accuracy and use of convincing perspective.[24] Some researchers suggest that this may be because autistic artists make no assumptions about the things they see in the world around them. Because they have not formed mental ideas of what is significant, they perceive all details as equally important. Instead of imposing visual or linguistic schema on the

world around them—a skill one needs to live in the world and conceptual-
ize rapidly—they absorb everything with the same high degree of inten-
sity.

Both mindblindness and the special talents of autistic people may reflect the same phenomenon—a situation in which the brain, for whatever
reason, is unable to process all the sensory information that is flowing into
it. For many autistic people, experiences that are normal for others, such
as being touched or listening to ordinary sounds, are painful. It may be
that autistic children throw tantrums and scream when they are touched
because to them touch is painful. They may be ultrasensitive to touch or
sound, since this neuronal system is hyperperceptive. Similarly, an autistic
child may exhibit an obsessive desire for routine, ritual, or sameness in his
or her environment, or become fixated on certain objects, in an attempt to
shut out the pain of an overload of sensory input. Another aspect of this
situation is that the autistic person does not perceive the world through abstract concepts as most of us do, but as an endless array of particulars to be
navigated through memorization and sorting-out of like images and experiences.

The autistic author Temple Grandin has explained that she has no abstract concept of "ship," but only images of every particular ship she has
ever encountered—the *Queen Mary,* the *Titanic,* and so on.[25] The flip side
of this working to compensate through endless sorting and processing of
particulars is that autistic people can develop remarkable skills in memorization, calculation, or technical artistry.

Strategies Used for the Management of Autism

I have studied many ways to help autistic children. My approach treats
the disorder at a core level, by addressing the root cause. In contrast, the
standard treatment for autism focuses mainly on the superficial aspects of
the disorder. The goal has been to *manage* rather than actually *treat* the
disorder. How do we manage autism? By reducing the symptoms of the
disorder through educational or behavioral therapies. Behavioral programs are meant to help children learn to reduce the number of tantrums,
and to become more communicative and less fearful. In some cases drugs
are administered to keep hyperactivity under control or help children
sleep. Special educational programs promote mental development.

These management strategies certainly can be helpful, and I believe they have an integral place in helping you reverse autism in your child. However, because the strategies do not address the underlying causes of autism, they are not likely to halt or reverse the progress of the condition. In my clinical experience, these strategies may help correct many of the manifestations of autism, such as lack of love and empathy, or the inability to abstract or socialize normally. Here's an overview of some of the most widespread therapeutic approaches to treating autism—educational and behavioral therapies, drugs, and nontraditional therapies.

Educational and Behavioral Therapies

When a child is diagnosed with autism, he or she will likely be enrolled in some form of speech, occupational, and/or play therapy. O. Ivar Lovaas of the University of California Los Angeles conducted a well-known study on this method, so one version of it has come to be known as Lovaas therapy. In 1987 Lovaas published his results, which showed that 47 percent of the children in the study, who were all under four years of age, were successfully "mainstreamed." Proponents of Lovaas have claimed that if you met these individuals now as teenagers, you would never know that anything had been wrong with them earlier in life. The program gained tremendous popularity after the 1993 publication of the book *Let Me Hear Your Voice,* by Catherine Maurice, in which she tells the story of how her two severely autistic children attained a complete recovery through the Lovaas program and other early intervention techniques. Although I have seen no legitimacy for this claim after meeting a number of youngsters who received Lovaas therapy, I do believe that it can help autistic children.

Drugs

I have been dismayed by reports of the alarming rise in prescriptions for medications intended to control behavioral disorders in children.[26] Some studies suggest that serotonin levels play a role in autism and the severity of its symptoms.[27] Serotonin transporter inhibitors appear to help reduce aggression and ritualistic behavior in many people.[28] Serotonin reuptake inhibitors have also proven helpful in some cases for reducing depression, panic disorder, and obsessive-compulsive disorder in autistic people—though in children they may be somewhat less effective.[29] Related research has also shown that when levels of tryptophan, a precursor to serotonin, are depleted, the central nervous system does not get enough serotonin, and stereotyped autistic behaviors may worsen.[30] According to one study, particular behaviors such as whirling, flapping, pacing, self-injurious behavior, rocking, and toe walking, as well as overall anxiety level, tend to worsen when tryptophan is depleted. This is probably related to diet, maldigestion, and malabsorption.[31]

Neuroleptic drugs such as haloperidol or trifluoperazine—which I consider dangerous—are also sometimes prescribed to reduce behavioral problems in children with PDD.[32] And in autistic children the drug sertraline may be used to help reduce anxiety, panic, and irritability related to changes of environment.[33]

At least one researcher has suggested that famotidine, an antihistamine that has been shown to relieve social deficit symptoms in schizophrenia, may also help autistic people. Histamine is a neurotransmitter that plays a role in inhibitory signals in the brain; blocking H2 receptors in the brain might result in less inhibited, more spontaneous and playful behavior.[34]

Nontraditional Therapies

Applied behavior analysis. Some children enter a special educational track, known as applied behavior analysis (ABA), though this program is not accepted by mainstream medicine. This program seeks to help autistic children develop socially useful skills. It involves highly intense and structured interactions with the child, including requests for the child to perform a task, and reinforcement from the teacher. This system is also known as intensive behavioral intervention (IBI). Teachers may interact one-on-one with autistic students anywhere from twenty to forty hours a week. This form of therapy asks the child to follow directions, perform simple tasks, or imitate the teacher. The child's behavior is then greeted with positive or (less often) negative reinforcement from the teacher. The idea is that tasks are broken down into small attainable parts. The goal is to develop skills that are prerequisites to language—attention, cooperation, and imitation. Acquiring new and constructive behaviors is emphasized. Later, children are taught skills that help them function both academically and socially.

Sensory processing therapies. This is a set of innovative treatment options for autistic people, based on the theory that autistic children and adults have a dysfunctional sensory system. This dysfunction is thought to be based in the central nervous system and brain. In particular, the three sensory systems that may be involved are tactile, vestibular (parts of the inner ear that detect movement and changes of position), and proprioceptive (subconscious awareness of body position through components of muscles, joints, and tendons). Sensory integration techniques such as auditory integration training (AIT) and pressure-touch can help reduce sensory overload.[35]

In AIT, which has proven to be particularly effective in reducing oversensitivity to sound, the subject listens to specially processed music that helps integrate his or her perception of sound frequencies. Bernard Rimland conducted a pilot study of AIT in seventeen autistic children aged four to twenty-one years. Eight children received AIT for ten days, while nine children listened to unprocessed music under identical conditions. Parents of the children in the AIT group noted decreases in repetitive behaviors, hyperactivity, and irritability, as well as improved attention.[36]

Facilitated communication (FC). This is a technique for helping autistic children to communicate through typing on a computer keyboard while being touched by an assistant.[37] However, there has been some debate over how much of the communication is coming from the autistic person, and how much from the assistant—since the assistant may appear to be facilitating the child's communication, while actually influencing it, whether consciously or unconsciously.

Secretin. The hormone secretin, secreted by the small intestine in response to food entering the digestive tract, has enjoyed controversial fame for the past several years. Secretin was accidentally "discovered" by Victoria Beck, the mother of an autistic child. In the course of routine tests for her child's gastrointestinal problems, Mrs. Beck found that secretin alleviated her son's diarrhea. Many parents have since reported that secretin has helped to alleviate their children's autistic symptoms, but the evidence remains largely anecdotal. No one knows how secretin works to help autistic patients, if in fact it does at all. To date, several double-blind clinical trials have cast doubt on the efficacy of secretin for treating autism.[38] For example, one randomized, double-blind, placebo-controlled study of twenty autistic people compared the effects of secretin to that of a placebo pill. Assessing the efficacy of both after either one month or two months, the researchers found no statistically significant difference between secretin and placebo.[39] Though secretin may help alleviate symptoms in some autistic children, the scientific evidence to date suggests it does not hold any promise in the treatment of autistic spectrum disorders.

Nutrition. Enzymes are used to help improve poor digestion and absorption, from which many autistic children suffer. Supplements and nutrients that may confer some benefit—based primarily on clinical observations of individual cases—include calcium, magnesium, vitamin A, and vitamin B_6; the amino acid tryptophan; essential fatty acids from fish oil or flaxseed oil; probiotics which may aid immune function in the gastrointestinal tract, and nutrition; and antifungals such as Diflucan and Nystatin. Ascorbic acid (vitamin C) may also help reduce symptoms in autistic children.[40] Melatonin, a neurohormone that also has antioxidant and immune-enhancing properties, has been used with some success as an antioxidant and to help autistic children sleep.[41]

Other therapies. A host of other alternative therapies have been used to treat autistic children and adults, including homeopathy, immunotherapy, and structural therapies such as massage, osteopathy, and craniosacral techniques. In later chapters, I will explain some of these therapies, and why I use them.

Breakthroughs in Early Diagnosis

In treating autism, early intervention is essential.[42] I believe this to be the case irrespective of the treatment approach used. And yet, early diagnosis of autism is notoriously difficult. Recent breakthroughs in the diagnosis of autism in very young infants suggest that the disease actually begins to manifest in fetal life, so it is most likely imperceptibly progressing long before it appears in a recognizable form, usually between ages two and three. Autopsies have shown that in autistic people the cells in the limbic regions of the brain, which mediate social behavior, are small and densely packed, suggesting that their early development was interrupted.[43] Recently, researchers have begun to develop a new set of diagnostic tools to help detect early signs of autism in toddlers, or even in very young infants.

Among the newest tools for early detection is a questionnaire designed for eighteen-month-old toddlers. Though autism does not usually appear in its full-blown form until somewhere between ages two and three, the questionnaire has proven to be somewhat successful in predicting which children are already exhibiting autistic tendencies at eighteen months. Simon Baron-Cohen and his colleagues at Cambridge University have developed an innovative screening tool to test for autistic symptoms in very young children. The "Checklist for Autism in Toddlers" (CHAT) consists of fourteen questions for parents and physicians of the child.

Using the CHAT diagnostic tool, four out of ninety-one eighteen-month-olds were identified who were diagnosed as autistic by age two and a half.[44]

One of the most promising methods for identifying autistic children in early infancy is a technique used to analyze infant movement, developed by Philip Teitelbaum and colleagues at the University of Florida. In a clinical study of seventeen autistic children, all seventeen showed movement abnormalities that could already be clearly identified at the age of four to six months.[45] These abnormalities include the shape of the mouth (called "Moebius syndrome") seen in the first few days after birth, as well as disturbances in milestones of development such as lying, righting, sitting, crawling, and walking.

Vision and hearing testing may prove to be another means of detecting autism early. In one study, infant hearing and vision were tested in a group of children who were subsequently diagnosed with autism, and compared with a group later diagnosed with nonspecific developmental delay, and a random control group. Four categories were investigated—motor, vision, hearing, and language/social skills—at ages six, twelve, and eighteen months. While the randomly sampled group had a low incidence of problems at each age, the learning-disabled group exhibited a sharp increase of abnormalities in all categories at twelve months. The autistic group had a selective increase in the social category alone at eighteen months.[46]

Children *diagnosed* with PDD have also been shown to exhibit impairments in social and communicative behaviors between twelve and thirty months of age, before they are finally diagnosed. Careful assessment of social interaction and communicative behaviors may help identify these children before the age of thirty months.[47]

Researchers are also looking for chemical clues that may predict later development of autism, so that fetuses can be tested for the disorder in utero, or babies at birth. One preliminary study of a mixed group of 246 teenagers whose blood had been sampled at birth identified a possible chemical marker for autism. The blood of the autistic or retarded children in the group showed elevated levels of four proteins related to brain development.[48] More work needs to be done in this area to determine whether a reliable blood test to predict autism can be developed.

Chapter 3

◆

The Ecology of Autism

When I was in medical school back in the 1960s, the disorder called autism was considered so rare that we paid it very little attention. Today, autism is no longer rare. In the summer of 2000, *Newsweek* announced that we now stand in the midst of an autism epidemic.[1] Only a decade ago, this condition of "mindblindness" was found in about 1 in 1,500 children in the United States. Most of the current estimates place the prevalence of autism at 1 in 1,000 U.S. children.[2] But a recently released report from the U.S. Centers for Disease Control and Prevention states that as many as 1 in every 500 U.S. children is affected by some form of autism.[3] This would represent a threefold jump in prevalence over a ten-year period.

Reports from many states do seem to suggest that autism is on the rise in the United States. A five-year study by the Department of Education documented a nationwide increase in the number of reported cases of autism of nearly 180 percent during the period of 1992 to 1997. Data collected by the California Department of Developmental Services show a 273 percent increase in the number of individuals receiving services for autism from 1987 to 1998.[4] Other states reporting a dramatic rise in autism rates in recent years include Connecticut, Indiana, Iowa, Maryland, Michigan, Nebraska, Nevada, New York, Ohio, Oregon, Pennsylvania, South Carolina, and Wisconsin. In the state of New York, for example, the number of autistic preschool and school-age children doubled from 1994 to 1998.[5]

At first glance, these trends seem quite frightening, particularly when you consider that the rising autism rates have greatly outpaced the increases in total population in those areas where new cases have been reported. I would urge caution however, when striving to interpret the numbers. Although I do believe there has been *some* increase in the rates of autism, the trends cited above are likely to reflect inflated estimates. A recent paper in *Pediatrics* convincingly argues that the purported jump in incidence "merely reflects the adoption of a much broader concept of autism, a recognition of autism among normally intelligent subjects, changes in diagnostic criteria, and an improved identification of persons with autism attributable to better services."[6] For example, changes in diagnostic concepts and definitions over the years have not been controlled in any of the surveillance efforts; thus, reports of autism rates today may reflect criteria that differ greatly from the old criteria. Along these lines, it is unclear whether the increases reflect only cases of *classic autism* or whether they fall into the broader category of *autistic spectrum disorders*—the broader definition would, of course, artificially inflate the numbers. Also, many autistic children are now diagnosed at a much earlier age, which naturally results in an increased number of reported cases.

At this time, it is unclear whether the number of cases of autism is indeed increasing, or whether the rise in diagnosed cases merely reflects a broadening of the definition of the disorder.[7] Another possibility may be that today's physicians may be more willing to diagnose autism than they once were. While autism used to be a hopeless diagnosis, today we know that early intervention can make a substantial difference in the outcome for an autistic child.[8] Most physicians, realizing this fact, may be less reluctant to report the disorder than they were in the past. But no one really knows.

Are the large increases in the prevalence of autism real, as some fervently claim, or are they mere statistical flukes for the reasons cited above? This much seems clear: The increased rates in many areas in the United States and elsewhere around the world are a matter of serious concern, if not a cause for alarm. The immense increases in some states are striking and should prompt more extensive research on the subject. My personal inclination is to err on the side of caution and assume there has been *some* increase in the incidence of autism. Such an increase might logically reflect an increase in pollution or toxic exposures—exposures that I believe play a major role in the genesis of autism. If this is shown to be the case, then we may very well have a national medical emergency on our hands, one that is likely to grow worse in the coming years unless major steps are taken to change the underlying environmental conditions that promote autism.

Figure 3-1

How a Genetically Based Disorder Becomes an "Epidemic"

Official estimates from the U.S. Centers for Disease Control indicate that autism has risen by approximately threefold over the past decade. Some scientists have questioned the veracity of the statistics, claiming that because we now know autism is caused by a genetic mutation, it can't really be an "epidemic." This view reflects a narrow understanding of genetics. It would be patently absurd, of course, to suggest that we have "an epidemic of genetic disease." Autistic people rarely if ever bear offspring: Only about 1 percent of autistic individuals will bear children. Thus, it is ludicrous to say that autism is increasing because more autistic individuals are passing on their aberrant genes. How, then, can a genetically based disease become an epidemic? The answer lies in the dynamic interaction between genes and xenobiotics (environmental pollutants), which are becoming more widespread over time, affecting ever-larger segments of the population. These pollutants damage the genes of perfectly normal individuals, either the parent or the developing fetus. The damage may occur prior to conception, during conception, soon after conception, or later in gestation. Such damage may continue to be inflicted throughout infancy. These are the critical windows during which xenobiotics can have the severest impact on the newborn infant.[9] The resulting genetic flaws are only the superficial cause of autism; the real cause is whatever created those flaws in the first place.

An Eco-Drama Surfaces in New Jersey

If my theory is correct, then we should expect to find higher concentrations of autistic cases in environmentally polluted areas—those areas affected by high levels of pollution. Numerous environmental pollutants are believed to be neurotoxins that can harm the developing fetus, infant, and young child.[10,11] For example, a pregnant mother's exposure to either mercury,[12] lead,[13] PCBs,[14] nicotine,[15] or various drugs (alcohol, cocaine, etc.)[16,17] may damage the fetal brain and predispose the child to behavioral problems. It is startling to note that a major action of many groups of pes-

ticides and chemical solvents is to disrupt neurological function.[18,19] All
neuroscientists understand that early life is a particularly vulnerable time
for the human nervous system. As I discussed in the first chapter, young
children living in polluted areas will be the first to manifest the adverse
impact of those pollutants on mental health.

To see how these connections relate to autism, consider the clustering
of autistic cases in Brick Township, a rural township located close to several
Superfund sites, approximately fifty miles south of Newark, New Jersey.
The possibility that pollution could be causing autism in Brick Township
came to light when a family with two autistic children (out of a total of
three) started asking questions about the extent of autism in the area. A
group of parents then began an informal surveillance effort, placing ads in
local newspapers to try to identify as many autistic cases as possible.
Based on the very large public response, the orchestrators of this informal
study calculated that the prevalence of autism in Brick Township was approximately three times the national average.[20]

In the 1990s, the U.S. Centers for Disease Control (CDC) and the
Agency for Toxic Substances and Disease Registry (ATSDR) carried out
an intensive investigation of autism rates and possible links with pollution
in Brick Township. On May 22, 2000, the reports from these agencies
were made public. They stated that the prevalence for strictly defined
autism was 4 per 1,000, and that prevalence for autistic spectrum disorders
was about 7 per 1,000.[21] These numbers are about four times the national
average. It seems likely that something in the environment has pushed the
rates upward. Many parents suspected that the local toxic landfill, which
had been in operation from 1949 through 1979, might account for the apparent increase in the risk of autism. During that period, the landfill had
been used for the disposal of municipal solid and liquid waste, sewage and
septic waste, and construction and commercial waste. An unknown number of labeled and unlabeled 55-gallon drums were also dumped in the
landfill, suggesting the presence of highly toxic pollutants. For this reason,
in 1982, the U.S. Environmental Protection Agency had added Brick
Township Landfill to its National Priority List.

In the course of their investigation, the CDC officials found that
municipal drinking water and well water contained three well-known toxic
pollutants—tetrachloroethylene, trichloroethylene, or trihalomethanes (THMs)—
at various times during the study period. According to the final Public
Health Assessment issued by the investigators, the total THM levels in the
municipal drinking water exceeded 80 parts per billion (ppb) several times

during the study period—a level that has been associated with DNA-damaging effects.[22] As I explain shortly, these genotoxic effects may provide the key to understanding the roots of autism. Such effects may have profound public health implications, since THMs often result from high chlorine levels in the drinking water, especially during the warmer seasons.

CDC officials also measured high levels of chemical and heavy metal pollutants in the groundwater beneath the landfill. They then argued, however, that residents would not have been exposed to the contaminated groundwater, because their drinking water came from the municipal water system. Similarly, they argued that any exposure to contaminated groundwater from irrigation wells near the site would not have been large or frequent enough to adversely affect the health of pregnant mothers or their offspring. The Public Health Assessment report also noted that a toxic "groundwater plume" has been spreading steadily in a southeastward direction, but then added, once again, that it "still does not present a public health hazard, because all residents in the area are on the municipal drinking water supply."[23]

Adopting a conservative position, the CDC investigators concluded that it "appeared unlikely" that the toxic chemicals found in the water supply were associated with autism in Brick Township. They reported "no clear pattern" linking location and timing of the autism cases with the high THM levels, or with levels of the other two toxic chemicals, tetrachloroethylene and trichloroethylene.

This conclusion—that there was no evidence of a link between the pollutants and autism in Brick Township—is clearly based on a narrow and speculative interpretation of the evidence. In truth, the CDC investigators do not *know* whether the high THM levels led to the increased risk of autism among these children. No one really knows, though that alone should be grounds for a more precautionary attitude. What's more, as I noted above, the CDC officials never actually measured levels of toxins in the body tissues of the autistic children and compared them to "normal" levels. (My research indicates they would have found very high levels of many toxins in the autistic children, and this would have led to radically different conclusions.)

I feel strongly that the CDC's investigation did not go far enough. Given that THMs are genotoxic, I'm more inclined to assume that the population is at risk for autism because of the high THM levels. Let's consider some of the recent findings concerning the potential risk of exposure to high THM levels:

1. **Potential link between THMs, neural tube defects, and autism**.
   In several studies, high THM levels were associated with at least a
   twofold increase in the risk of neural tube defects.[24,25,26] Strikingly,
   these THM levels were well within the range of those levels found
   in the Brick Township municipal water supply. This is important,
   since a neural tube defect—that is, failure of the tube to close up
   properly during embryonic development—may represent the initial
   brain injury in the genesis of autism, as the CDC officials acknowledged in their final report.[27,28,29]

2. **Potential link between THMs, chromosomal damage, and autism**.
   As I discussed earlier, chromosomal damage plays a predisposing
   role in autism. Laboratory studies have shown that THMs can cause
   chromosomal abnormalities and DNA damage.[30] Two recent reports
   from Canada suggest that chromosomal abnormalities increase in
   infants whose mothers drink water high in THMs (chloroform) during or prior to pregnancy.[31,32] These studies were specifically designed to test the potential impact of THM-tainted drinking water
   on birth defects and other adverse birth outcomes.

3. **Potential link between THMs, low birthweight, and autism**.
   Nearly one out of every three infants of extremely low birthweight
   is at high risk for autism, mental retardation, cerebral palsy, or other
   serious neurodevelopmental problems.[33] Small birth size[34,35] and
   spontaneous abortion (miscarriage)[36] have been associated with high
   levels of THMs in drinking water. A 1998 report from David Savitz
   and colleagues at the University of North Carolina points to a "potentially important relation between third trimester exposure to trihalomethanes and retarded fetal growth."[37]

4. **Potential link between THMs, neurotoxicity, and autism**. In
   1982, *Environmental Health Perspectives* reported on research
   showing that exposure to various THMs resulted in behavioral abnormalities in laboratory mice. The researchers observed these
   aberrant behaviors, or "behavioral toxicity," in the mice offspring
   following extensive exposure to THMs during pregnancy.[38] Other
   rodent studies have demonstrated toxic effects of THMs on both the
   liver and kidneys.[39]

As you can see, substantial evidence now suggests that congenital anomalies can result from exposure to higher-than-normal levels of THMs. Whether such anomalies lead to autism remains an open question. At this juncture, however, I would recommend that public health officials base their recommendations for the people of Brick Township on the *precautionary principle*.[40] This means they should take every conceivable measure to reduce the population's risk of exposure to THMs and possibly other forms of pollution in the drinking water. Given the totality of scientific evidence to date, I propose that the high THM levels alone could have damaged the DNA of parents who then gave birth to children with damaged livers—children who then became autistic.

The federal Centers for Disease Control, based here in Atlanta, devoted considerable time, money, and energy to investigating the reasons for the excess of autistic cases in Brick Township. At one point I spoke with a CDC official who had read my paper on autism and environmental toxicity, published in *Toxicology & Industrial Health*.[41] The research presented in that paper clearly revealed the environmental connection, showing extremely high levels of pollutants in autistic children. There were several genotoxic chemicals that might account for the high rates of autism at Brick Township. It is disturbing to me that the CDC and ATSDR investigators never bothered to measure tissue levels of various chemical toxins and heavy metals in children living in these areas, and then compare the results of autistic to nonautistic children.

Other kinds of learning disabilities also appear to be clustered in *environmentally toxic* areas. An unusually high rate of learning disabilities and emotional problems among families in Anniston, Alabama, has recently been linked to the polychlorinated biphenyls (PCBs) emitted by the Monsanto pharmaceutical plant in the town for the past several decades.[42] We should not dismiss such associations as flukes or aberrations, but instead consider how they may be affecting larger segments of the population, obviously in a more diffuse manner.

I find it entirely plausible that the poisons in our air and water supplies every day are responsible for the rising incidence of both autistic disorders and learning disabilities among children today. The epidemiological and clinical evidence shows a clear link between exposure to environmental toxins and developmental abnormalities in the human brain.[43] Keep in mind that the nervous systems of the developing fetus and young infant are particularly vulnerable to the effects I've just described.[44] We have only skimmed the surface in our understanding of these xenobiotic threats to the young child's brain.

The question of multiple chemical exposures represents an extremely complex challenge to those of us investigating the potential adverse effects of pollution on behavioral development. Nevertheless, studies of both animals and humans have repeatedly shown that prenatal exposure to heavy metals, synthetic chemicals, and drugs can collectively impair the neurobehavioral development of the offspring.[45] Moreover, specific combinations of metals, solvents, and pesticides can contribute to problems in learning, memory, and behavior.[46]

In any case, the research suggests that some, or perhaps all, of the autistic children in Brick Township were the victims of *multiple chemical and heavy metal exposures*—not just the THM issue I highlighted earlier. This must be considered a distinct possibility, one that has at least one historic precedent. In 1975, the National Institute of Health did a study of 55,908 pregnancies that found a significant correlation between women who worked in occupations that involved handling various chemicals, and giving birth to autistic children.[47] Similar findings were reported in a study at the Children's Brain Disorder Clinic in Washington, D.C.[48] Oddly, however, no follow-up studies were ever conducted.

The search for a cause of autism is gaining urgency as the incidence of the disease continues to rise. My own research suggests, again, that many chemicals and heavy metals in the environment can promote neurodevelopmental disabilities, including the whole range of autism spectrum disorders. As our environment becomes more polluted, I predict that we will see more birth defects, behavioral abnormalities, and cases of autism in the coming years. We should be doing everything in our power to safeguard future generations against this terrible prospect.

It is my hope that investigations such as that of Brick Township will help bring more serious attention to this issue. Once the xenobiotic link is firmly established, the next step is to unravel the mechanisms by which such environmental hazards damage the developing brain and nervous system to cause autism. Only then can we begin to reverse the process.

Autism's Association with Other Medical Conditions

Over the past several decades, ever since Kanner first identified the disorder called autism, there has been an ongoing effort to pinpoint risk factors and causes of the disease, with one theory after another gaining credence and then disappearing into oblivion. When autism was thought to be a psychiatric disorder, it was often attributed to psychological factors, such as humorless and perfectionistic parenting. Once it was established that autism has a neurological basis,[49,50] researchers turned their attention to identifying its specific neurological causes. Roughly a third of all cases of autism are associated with other medical conditions that are suspected links to the pathogenesis of the disorder[51]—but this knowledge has not brought us any closer to a cure.

Over the past forty years, scientists have linked autism with many etiologies, including phenylketonuria,[52,53,54] histidinemia,[55,56] heparin-n-sulfatase deficiency,[57] tuberous sclerosis,[58] fragile X syndrome,[59,60] rubella,[61,62] cytomegalovirus,[63,64] celiac disease,[65] herpes simplex, and a host of other possible risk factors.[66,67,68,69,70,71,72,73] Other factors related to autism include low birthweight and perinatal or postnatal trauma or insults.[74,75] Gastrointestinal disorders such as reflux esophagitis and malabsorption likely also contribute—albeit indirectly—to the behavioral problems of some autistic children.[76]

Epilepsy is also associated with autism, and may explain some fluctuations in impairment of language, cognitive, and motor skills.[77] About one third of children with autism will experience at least two unprovoked epileptic seizures by the time they reach adulthood.[78] In the 1970s, reports of a correlation between epilepsy and autism helped overturn the belief that autism was the result of inept parenting. Some researchers suspect that epilepsy may cause autism and severe language impairment, while others point to underlying brain abnormalities as the cause for both autism and language deficits.[79]

Research on Environmental Contributors to Autism

Since 1976, when Spence described autism as having polygenetic characteristics, the theory of polygenetic spontaneous mutation has become the most widely accepted causal theory of autism. Indeed, there is well-known evidence for the role of genetic factors in the disorder. Studies show that identical twins have a 90 percent concordance rate for the disorder, while fraternal twins show only a 25 percent concordance rate.[80] The fact that there is a much higher incidence of autism among males also points to some underlying genetic factor, although we have not yet found a specific mechanism to explain this phenomenon.[81,82,83,84]

As I noted above, genetic theories do not go far enough to really explain the epidemic of autism we are witnessing. Although the autistic phenotype runs in families with varying degrees of severity, it is hard to imagine that "autistic genes" could be passed on in such high numbers, especially since so few autistic people bear offspring. The number of new cases appears to be rising too rapidly to be explained simply as the result of a genetic aberration. Genotoxic damage from free radicals and other so-called environmental insults are the more plausible cause. For example, mothers who consume alcohol during pregnancy may unwittingly heighten the risk of autism and other neurodevelopmental disorders in their offspring.[85,86,87] These reports focused on a relatively small number of cases, however, and the findings need to be verified in large clinical trials.

Among the more striking examples of a genotoxic insult leading to autism is a pregnant woman's exposure to the (now banned) drug thalidomide. In 1995, a group of ophthalmologists reported on a Swedish population of thalidomide survivors.[88] Out of eighty-six people who had been exposed to thalidomide in the womb, four were autistic. All four were among the fifteen cases who had early exposure to the drug, between days 20 and 24 after conception. No cases of autism were identified outside of this narrow window of exposure. The research to date suggests that thalidomide exposure during this period of embryonic development can result in a fiftyfold increased risk of autism compared to children not exposed to thalidomide.

A small follow-up study by the same researchers seemed to confirm the effect of this prenatal toxic insult to the brain.[89] Pregnant rats exposed to valproic acid, a chemical that interrupts the closing of the neural tube, gave birth to offspring whose brain tissues were altered in ways similar to those observed in postmortem studies of autistic individuals (several serious birth defects—spina bifida, anencephaly, and encephalocele—are also known to result from failure of neural tube closure during the first month of embryonic development.)[90] It is possible that prenatal exposure to many different substances could account for the neural tube defects that predispose some infants to autism. These include the following vast groups of xenobiotics: organic solvents such as many cleaning agents; x-rays and other forms of ionizing radiation; pesticides and other agricultural chemicals; water nitrates; mercury and other heavy metals; and water disinfection by-products, such as the THMs I highlighted in the Brick

Township story.[91] With regard to pesticides, women who live near pesticide-treated agricultural areas have a 50 percent increased risk of giving birth to infants with neural tube defects; the risk is 60 percent *higher* for pregnant women who have professionals apply pesticides in the home environment.[92]

Even nutritional supplements can be problematic when used irresponsibly before and during pregnancy. A deficiency of either folic acid or zinc during pregnancy may *promote* neural tube defects, while an excess (megadose) of vitamin A can be equally harmful.[93,94] Megadosing with vitamin A during pregnancy has been associated with birth defects, which is why the FDA routinely advises pregnant women to limit their vitamin A intake from liver or supplements to 5,000 IU per day. A recent clinical trial indicates, however, that much higher vitamin A intakes, in the range of 50,000 to 300,000 IU per day, are probably safe for the majority of pregnant women.[95] My preference would be to set the gestational limit at 50,000 IU, given that vitamin A at doses easily obtained from supplements could, in theory, potentiate the toxic effects of some xenobiotics on fetal development.[96]

Another possible way to curb the threat of neural tube defects is to use antioxidant supplements. Diabetic mothers or women suffering from temporarily high blood sugar (diabetic pregnancy) may be at especially high risk of giving birth to children with such defects. It is thought that the high blood sugar levels lead to increased oxidative stress, which then promotes birth defects. This is why obstetricians encourage such women to carefully control blood sugar levels during pregnancy.[97] A recent laboratory study showed that lipoic acid reduced the incidence of neural tube defects in pregnant diabetic rats.[98] This is consistent with studies of other antioxidants that have been shown to lower the rate of congenital malformations induced by high glucose levels, including vitamin E,[99] N-acetyl cysteine (NAC),[100] inositol,[101] zinc,[102] and superoxide dismutase.[103] To reduce oxidative stress during pregnancy, taking a combination of antioxidants would seem to be a good idea not only for diabetic women, but also for overweight women and those with a history of toxic exposures.

I believe that a combination of xenobiotic damage to the nervous system, a genetic predisposition to liver abnormalities, and an immune system compromised by toxic overload, together produce the disorder called autism. The recent controversy over a possible link between the measles-mumps-rubella (MMR) vaccine and autism affords a valuable opportunity to elucidate this view.

The Vaccine Controversy

Concerned parents and antivaccine activists point to two dangers that vaccines might pose, factors they see as possible causes of autism. One is the introduction of a live virus into an infant's body, and the other is the use, until recently, of a mercury-containing preservative called thimerosal in many vaccines. I would like to briefly address both these issues. While I do not believe that vaccines cause autism, they may in some cases trigger or push over the edge a case where a child's immune system is already compromised.

A researcher named Andrew Wakefield, of the Royal Free Hospital, UK, is largely responsible for the recent surge of controversy over a possible causal link between the MMR vaccine and autism. In 1998, he published a well-known study linking autism to intestinal abnormalities in twelve children, possibly caused by the MMR vaccine.[104] Based on this study, Wakefield suggested that the vaccine in its current form should be discontinued, and its components introduced separately. Wakefield has since coined a name for this autism–gut virus combination he has identified, "autistic enterocolitis."[105] He and his colleagues later claimed that in one study they discovered measles virus in the gastrointestinal tracts of twenty-four out of twenty-five children with autism, compared with one of fifteen controls.[106]

Wakefield's theory of a causal link between the MMR vaccine and autism, however, has since been almost totally discredited. The following year another research group from the same institution performed a study that found no causal connection between the vaccine and autism.[107] Several studies have since failed to find a causal link between MMR and autism. Another study found no association between inflammatory bowel disease and autism among children immunized with the MMR vaccine.[108] Furthermore, Wakefield's research methods have been widely criticized.[109]

I agree with the conclusion that there is no direct causal link between the MMR vaccine and autism. First, the MMR is administered at age twelve to fifteen months. Most parents of autistic children first identify abnormalities in their child's behavior around the age of eighteen months. This temporal association may or may not indicate a cause-and-effect relationship; in all likelihood, it is just a coincidence. Many children have developed autism without ever having received the vaccine, and autistic symptoms may occur in infants before they reach one year of age, i.e., before they would be vaccinated. Furthermore, there is no evidence that the live virus in the MMR vaccine, or in any other vaccine, can "overwhelm" the immune system of a child, one of the central theories of antivaccine activists. In fact, vaccines tax the immune system far less than natural diseases do—although much depends on the relative strength of the child's immune system at the time of vaccination.

I do not doubt that Dr. Wakefield did find measles virus in the colons of the autistic children he has studied. Children who receive the MMR vaccine are given live measles virus at age twelve to eighteen months. Their immune systems are incapable of eradicating the virus completely once it enters the body. Autistic children have low levels of natural killer (NK) cell activity and are basically immune-suppressed to begin with. This is most likely due to an overload of immune-suppressing toxins such as mercury, lead, and others. The measles virus, as well as other viruses, will flourish in an environment where the immune system cannot eradicate it. This is the reason we find measles virus growing in the colons of these autistic children.

Does this mean that the measles virus is the cause of autism? No, of course not. It is a "side chain reaction" because of a dysfunctional immune system. The real question is why the immune system in these children is so weakened in the first place. The fact that all of the autistic children I have treated show dangerously high levels of a variety of harmful environmental toxins is an important clue to understanding this phenomenon.

Thimerosal may have played a larger role in triggering autism in some children. I do not view it as the "cause" of autism either, but as a possible link, a factor that may tip a situation verging on toxic overload into a state of crisis. Thimerosal is not used in the MMR vaccine, but it has been used in several other common vaccines, including hepatitis B, Hib, and DTP. It is incredible that no study has ever been done to test the safety of using thimerosal in children's vaccines, despite the fact that it has been in use for the past seventy years.[110] Though the evidence remains anecdotal, there are many reported cases in which parents of autistic children said they were normal until receiving thimerosal-containing vaccinations, particularly DTP.[111]

Thimerosal was widely used until 1999, when the FDA and the American Academy of Pediatrics finally determined that many of the vaccinated babies were receiving levels of mercury that exceeded government safety guidelines.[112] In fact, in many cases these levels were twice as high as what the EPA had deemed safe for young children.[113] By early 2001, thimerosal had been completely phased out of use in vaccines, although it can still be found in vaccines that are on the shelves in pharmacies or doctors' offices. Until 1999, no one had really stopped to consider that the levels of mercury deemed safe in these vaccines were *adult* levels. The same amount of mercury that might be safe for an adult could damage the developing nervous system of an infant.

It is no coincidence that autism and mercury poisoning share many characteristic symptoms—speech, language, and social deficits; motor disorders and cognitive impairments; and even unique behavioral symptoms such as hand flapping, toe walking, and unusual responses to noise.[114,115,116] Many cases of *idiopathic* autism (that is, autism of unknown etiology) may in fact have been induced by exposure to the mercury in thimerosal. At the same time, thimerosal probably triggers autism only in children who are already susceptible to its toxic effects. This susceptibility might be due to both genetic and nongenetic factors, including the total mercury burden from the mother and from air, water, and food.

A Whirlwind Tour of the Biology of Autism

Brain Abnormalities

The past five decades of research into autism have left medical science with a rather fragmented view of the root causes of this disease. Autism has been linked to a functional deficit in the cerebral cortex, the large frontal part of the brain where complex information processing takes place. Our highly active cortex is among the primary physical features that set us apart from other members of the animal kingdom. A healthy, fully functioning cerebral cortex enables us to enjoy a vast range of cognitive processes as well as complex social behaviors. PET scans in autistic kids show a decreased uptake of glucose in the cortical and subcortical regions of the brain. Higher-order memory, attention, language, auditory information processing, and conceptual reasoning ability are all compromised to some degree in autistic individuals.[117]

In addition to problems with cortical activity, autopsy specimens of autistic persons show certain abnormalities (such as a stunting of the dendritic tree) in the limbic system,[118] the part of the brain associated with emotions. This basic aberration may account for a great deal of emotional distress in these children. Autistic children also exhibit abnormalities in the cerebellum, the part of the brain serving to coordinate voluntary movements and balance in humans.

Pathological studies of young brains have demonstrated that the exact timing of toxic exposures is of the essence in the incipient development of autism. As I noted previously, the fetal brain is highly vulnerable to toxic insults from the mother's bloodstream, and the third trimester appears to be a critical time for autism-related brain injury. There is, however, some controversy on the latter point. As I noted earlier, a Swedish study found that thalidomide exposure in the first trimester—particularly between days 20 and 24 of pregnancy—led to a high rate of autism.[119] This effect on the brain may be traced to a shortening of the brain stem.[120]

At the present time, our neuropathological studies of brains of autistic people are limited, with fewer than thirty-five brains studied (none with modern techniques). Nonetheless, these studies do show subtle prenatal neuronal maldevelopment in the cerebellum and certain limbic structures.[121] Indeed, autism has been associated with a developmental delay during gestation or early life, a late maturation of the central nervous system.[122] The brains tend to be larger than average; they also exhibit smaller than normal, more tightly packed cells in some cerebellar nuclei and limbic structures, and a reduced number of Purkinje cells and granular cells in parts of the cerebellar cortex, including the amygdala and hippocampus, suggesting defective development during gestation.[123] Intriguingly, several of the primary brain changes have been replicated in laboratory animals born to mothers that had been exposed to toxic chemicals during pregnancy.[124]

Autistic people also exhibit abnormal or insufficient blood flow to certain areas of the brain. One study showed that a group of thirty moderately to severely mentally retarded autistic patients had significantly lower than normal blood flow in the right temporal lobe (base inferior areas), occipital lobes, thalami, and left basal ganglia.[125] Neuroimaging has shown abnormalities of blood circulation in the medial prefrontal cortex and anterior cingulate gyrus, which are thought to be related to cognitive deficits, and also abnormal blood flow in the right medial temporal lobe, associated with the obsessive desire for sameness.[126] These patterns of blood flow suggest possible locations of brain function that are associated with the abnormal behavior patterns we find in autism.

Altered immunity and Other Theories

Numerous theories have been proposed to explain the *etiology,* or cause and development, of autism. Many of these theories center around peculiar responses by the immune system. For example, a heightened susceptibility to yeast infections and extreme reactions to gluten peptides are both associated with autistic tendencies. Allergic reactions to foods such as wheat, corn, tomatoes, sugar, mushrooms, and dairy products may contribute to many of the behavioral problems seen in autistic individuals.[127] Under healthy conditions, the immune system keeps foreign substances and microbes out of the body in a peaceful and efficient manner. Not so, ostensibly, with a great many autistic individuals.

In short, there is ample evidence that immune dysfunction is somehow linked to the development of autistic characteristics.[128] In many autistic individuals, the immune system is simply off kilter. This is evidenced by a number of factors, including certain changes in the function of NK cells and T cells,[129,130] as well as decreased response to mitogens,[131,132] antibodies to myelin basic protein (the myelin sheath protects nerve fibers),[133] and various abnormalities in cytokine production.[134] Cytokines are a vast group of proteins that carry messages between immune cells and between these cells and other tissues.

In my view, however, the immune system *per se* is not the central problem. Rather, it should be considered a side issue, albeit one well worth addressing. Let us consider a certain group of immune cells known as natural killer (NK) cells, which display a wide variety of immune activities. In autistic children, the activity of NK cells is often compromised.[135,136] The same is often true in other autistic spectrum disorders, such as Rett syndrome.[137] Immunologists who are well versed in toxicology know that toxins such as mercury vapors can heavily suppress NK activity.[138] When somebody is under chronic toxic stress—perhaps due to heavy metals or petrochemicals that have accumulated in their fatty tissue—NK activity is bound to be low. It's an immunological given.

Some research has shown a hyperactive and misdirected immune response in children with autism and other neurological disorders, and this may ultimately help us better understand their etiology. One manifestation of the aberrant immune response, seen in children with either autism or Landau-Kleffner syndrome, is a greater frequency of serum antibodies to brain endothelial cells and nuclei in these children compared with normal children.[139] Children with autism also often have antibodies against myelin basic protein, which would also suggest an autoimmune response.[140] The presence of such antibodies suggests that autoimmunity, an abnormal reaction to one's own body tissues, may play a central role in the development of these disorders.

I will discuss the nature of this heightened immune response in more detail in Chapter 5, "Understanding the Autism Complex," in which I lay out the details of my theory of the pathogenesis of this disease. This research is extremely important because approximately half of the autistic children I have studied exhibit a particular autoimmune process that attacks the brain. (See my discussion of our fourth study's findings in Chapter 1.) These patterns of immune response can be clearly related to *toxic effects on the immune system*. The immune system reactions that have been documented are related to the xenobiotic effects of lead, mercury, and other heavy metals and chemical toxins. This fits with everything I have discovered in treating autistic children. In all cases, they have been exposed to high levels of environmental toxins, which their bodies are trying unsuccessfully to deal with. This is the direction we must look for further insight into the pathogenesis of this disease.

Research already shows that this immune connection may have therapeutic relevance to autism. For example, opioid-immune interactions are known to be abnormal in many autistic children. In one study, autistic children were treated with the potent opiate antagonist naltrexone, and this resulted in a number of behavioral improvements. The positive behavioral changes were accompanied by specific improvements in immune system functioning. Specifically, the ratios of T-helper to T-suppressor cells became normalized, and NK cell activities increased as the levels of natural opiates (e.g., beta-endorphins) decreased.[141] The burgeoning field of psychoneuroimmunology has established numerous connections between the brain and the immune system.

A proponent of the nutritional approach, Dr. Michael Goldberg, espouses a combination of a dairy-free diet and a special vitamin supplement which he believes can help rectify the autistic's dysregulated immune system. He reports that additional benefits may accrue with the use of an amino acid supplement called dimethylglycine as well as various antiyeast and behavior modification strategies. Using these strategies, Goldberg claims that children can recover normal functioning; however, he has never conducted any clinical studies to back up these claims.[142] My own findings indicate, moreover, that these strategies do not address the underlying processes that drive autism and thus have limited therapeutic benefit.

Regarding the peptide connection, we do know that some autistic children—not necessarily a majority—have increased levels of peptides in their urine. Peptides are fragments of protein, and ordinarily they are broken down further into amino acids. These poorly digested proteins include casein from cow's milk products, as well as gluten from wheat products. An influx of these peptides could, in theory, have toxic consequences in the brain. About 50 percent of autistic patients have highly permeable intestinal tracts, enabling these protein fragments to more readily enter the bloodstream.[143] Autistics often show deficiencies in the IgA antibody system of the digestive tract, the antibody system that normally keeps food antigens (foreign proteins) from entering the bloodstream via the intestinal lining.[144] When you remove dairy and wheat from the diet, these patients typically get better.

Besides the "leaky gut" syndrome seen in some autistic people, another explanation for the abnormally high levels of peptides is a lack of key enzymes known as peptidases, which break down peptides into amino acids in the small intestine. This problem can be traced, at least in part, to low dietary levels of the trace element zinc. Many autistic patients show low zinc levels in their red blood cells. Simply by supplementing the diet with zinc, many of these children begin to show signs of improvement, both behaviorally and immunologically.

In addition, however, our clinical observations indicated that these children often show a very low production of pancreatic enzymes. The pancreas must be functioning normally to ensure the complete breakdown of proteins in the intestine. If you damage the pancreas, these enzymes just won't be produced in sufficient quantity. In this case, a specific type of nutritional intervention is needed to support the pancreas and get it functioning at a normal level again.

A second common problem we have seen in these individuals is abnormal kidney function. The kidney contains millions of fine filtering structures known as nephrons. The tubules within nephrons are at times damaged in autistic individuals, resulting in an inability to *reabsorb* zinc and other essential nutrients, including specific amino acids, peptides, and neurotransmitters. For this reason, autistic children may often lose large amounts of essential minerals and trace elements through the urine. Injury to the renal tubules has been shown to result from early-life exposure to toxic chemicals and heavy metals.

Third, these children may actually require additional amounts of the very same micronutrients they are losing through the urine. It is well established that psychological stress can increase the brain's requirement for zinc and other elements. If autistic people become zinc deficient, they typically need to be supplemented beyond the level normally considered "adequate" for a healthy child.

Like the measles virus found in the colons of the autistic children in Andrew Wakefield's study, these are all side reactions to a body damaged by toxic metals and chemicals. The peptides from gluten and casein are the result of poor digestion due to low zinc levels, which I have found in at least half of the autistic children coming to my Atlanta clinic. Similarly, free radical damage to the pancreas leads to a lack of pancreatic enzymes. In the past, this certainly has been shown in scientific studies where xenobiotics caused free radical damage to the pancreas.

Detoxication is an extremely delicate process, and if either phase is out of balance with the other, the result may be the production of highly toxic chemicals that can have an adverse effect on the brain and nervous system. If phase I is overactive in relation to phase II, this can lead to a "backup" of chemicals in the body and the production of toxic metabolites (free radical compounds) that do not easily find their way out of the body. If phase I is operating efficiently but phase II is not, this can lead to the production of free radicals which can inflict oxidative damage throughout the body, as well as an accumulation of toxic chemicals which become absorbed in the body's fatty tissues. There is good evidence to suggest that genetic abnormalities may cause these problems with the chemistry of detoxication.

In children whose liver function is already out of balance, poor nutrition makes the problem still worse. Their bodies are even less able to cope with these toxins. Thus, their brain dysfunction tends to become worse over time. I will draw on a growing body of evidence to support this provocative theory in the next few chapters of this book.

Autistic Genes?

It is clear that there is a strong genetic component to autism. We know, for instance, that autism is very common in identical twins, while it is surprisingly rare for fraternal twins to both develop the disease. There is a 90 percent rate of concordance for autism—though possibly of different levels of severity—among identical twins, with a 25 percent concordance among same-sex fraternal twins.[146] In families with one autistic child, there is a 3 to 8 percent risk of recurrence.[147] Asperger's syndrome, too, appears to run in families—often at least one parent of an affected child also has the disorder.

Males are affected with autism four times more often than females, apparently because the genes associated with autism are sex-linked. Certain chromosomal abnormalities have been clearly associated with infantile autism.[148] The types of abnormalities may be associated with degrees of cognitive delay, though not necessarily with autistic severity.[149]

Before going further, keep in mind that these genetic abnormalities do not simply arise out of nowhere, and they are not inherited or passed on from one generation to the next. Rather, the evidence to date strongly indicates that the genetic flaws result from genotoxic injury—damage to either the sperm, the egg, or the developing embryo, or some combination thereof. (Please refer to the previous chapter for a more detailed discussion of these relationships.)

Abnormalities inherited from the mother on chromosome 15 are the most common genetic link with autism.[150] Fragile X syndrome is a prevalent cause of mental retardation in males, but most people with fragile X are not autistic. The fragile X chromosome abnormality is associated with autism anywhere between 0 to 53 percent of the time. Its incidence is roughly equal to that among mentally retarded males—suggesting that it is not an aberration that increases the risk of autism over that of mental retardation.[151] It accounts for only 1 to 2.5 percent of people with autistic spectrum disorders.[152] One study found that genes on the X chromosome were not responsible for any moderate to strong effect causing autism, but the authors suggested that genes on the X chromosome might be responsible for a "minor" degree of causal influence.[153] Another group of researchers, however, suggested that this X chromosome influence is not so minor at all, but may in fact explain much if not all of the approximately seventy-five-fold increased risk of autism among siblings of autistic children.[154]

The important point is that genes do not function in isolation from the environment. In fact, the genetic material (both DNA and RNA) is constantly interacting with the biochemical milieu surrounding and pervading each living cell. Environmental factors are needed to trigger the expression of certain genes, and may alter the genes themselves, resulting in mutations (genotoxicity) and in the abnormal production of proteins needed for healthy functioning of the whole human being.

Allow me to summarize the key points about the genetic aspects of autism. Clearly, the rise in the incidence of autism is too steep to be attributed to a series of genetic aberrations passed on from one generation to the next. Genetic factors interact constantly with environmental factors. The genotoxic influence of an increasingly polluted environment is the only plausible way to explain this ominous epidemic.

A Marriage of Genotoxicity and Neurotoxicity

The influence of the environment on autism is beyond dispute. As a 1999 report in the *Journal of Psychiatry & Neuroscience* notes, "the prevailing view is that autism is caused by a pathophysiologic process arising from the interaction of an early environmental insult and a genetic predisposition."[155] We see the environmental connection played out in the global distribution of autism. Rates of the disorder are highest in developed countries where the nuclear family and a high degree of mobility (geographical and economic) predominate.[156,157,158] These Westernized countries—Japan and the United States, for example—have one environmental variable in common: increasing exposure to neurotoxicants in and around the home and workplace. This explains why growing up in the city is generally associated with an increased risk of neurodevelopmental disorders compared to growing up outside the city—independent of any exposure to drugs in the womb.[159] It also explains why we have begun to see clusters of autism in environmentally sensitive areas, such as Brick Township.

Autism appears to arise from the convergence of genetic defects (again, due to genotoxic injury), defects in liver detoxication, and toxic insults to the developing brain and nervous system. By "developing brain and nervous system" I am referring to damage that could occur either in the womb or soon after birth. My own speculation is that at least 90 percent of autistic cases result from haphazard toxic damage to the neurons (neurotoxicity) in the infant's brain. Such toxic damage could take the form of environmental toxins, free radicals, auto-antibodies, and inflammatory reactions that result in yet more free radicals. For this to occur, however, there must also be a genetic defect in liver detoxication. Such defects, already clearly identified, result in abnormal levels of key detoxifying liver enzymes.[160,161,162]

The reason for the wide spectrum of autistic manifestations relates to which amounts of which toxins cause injury to the brain, and when and where in the brain exactly the damage occurs. This is probably true not only of autism but of a whole range of developmental problems in children. According to a recent study from the National Academy of Sciences, a combination of neurotoxins and genetic factors may account for nearly 25 percent of developmental problems in children.[163] I suspect this number is actually much higher.

In our recent paper for the *Journal of Toxicology & Industrial Health,* Dr. Cantor and I conclude that "a chronic toxicological mechanism is occurring in autism" and moreover that "autism may begin as early as the fetal development period. This is a time when the central nervous system is quite vulnerable to influences from the external environment because of the lack of a protective blood brain barrier."[164] The most crucial window of development—when toxins can do the most damage—is during fetal life.

The prenatal developing brain is constantly becoming more complex— adding new cells, connections, special areas, and complex networks of cellular communication. Anything that disrupts this normal brain development may have effects on the sensory, social, language, and mental functions of the fetus and the newborn. I believe that during this most vulnerable period the fetus may become burdened with environmental neurotoxins of all sorts, and this sequence of events leads to the autistic spectrum of illnesses.

In the fetus (as well as in the mother), the liver has a limited capacity to detoxify lipophilic chemicals that enter the fetus's body. These toxic agents thus have easy access to neurons and dendritic processes. As the central nervous system is exposed to these toxic agents, the brain of the fetus develops microscopic pathology.

Studies have shown that exposure to toxic environmental chemicals (xenobiotics) is a significant characteristic of a large proportion of families of autistic children.[165,166] Even though the brain has a protective barrier (the blood-brain barrier) that shields it from exposure to harmful toxins from the environment, some toxins do get through. Chemicals could get to the fetus through the mother's bloodstream or after birth directly into the body through the skin, lungs, or gastrointestinal tract. It is well known that chronic neurotoxic effects are associated with physiological changes in the structure of the nervous system.[167,168] Such changes could lead to the kinds of abnormalities often found in autistic children, including damage to dendrites, neurons, axons, myelin, and myelin-forming cells. Autistic children may suffer damage to their developing nervous systems due to an interaction among these toxic agents, the immune system, and direct or free radical injuries—a combination that subjects the central nervous system to chronic low-level neurotoxicity.

Because of the nature of these impairments, if the autistic disorder is caught before age three, I believe we can predict a probable high percentage of improvement in cognitive and emotional functioning. This is because the brain has tremendous "plasticity" before we begin our fourth year of life. Plasticity refers to the brain's capacity to change in significant ways in response to early-life experiences. We now know that the brain's capacity in this regard is not genetically determined or fixed at birth. The brain itself can be altered—or guided in its development—with appropriately timed, intensive intervention.

I will return to this point again and again throughout this book because it is applicable to a wide range of mental health issues. The experiences that fill a baby's first days, months, and years have a decisive impact on the architecture of the brain, as well as on the nature and extent of the individual's adult capacities. During these first few years, millions of neuronal connections are being made and remade on a day-to-day basis. Some brain cells are literally "turned on" by a particular experience; many new connections among brain cells are formed, while existing connections can be further strengthened.

This early-life brain plasticity has profound implications for children with autistic tendencies. It means that severely injured brains—injury resulting from a toxic environmental insult—can reestablish normal functioning in a very short time with the proper attention.

There is also, however, a more disturbing aspect to the brain's plasticity. The changeable nature of the brain means that there are times when negative experiences or the wrong types of environmental exposures are more likely to have serious and sustained effects. The infant's brain is highly vulnerable to toxins during the first three years.[169] This includes early exposure to nicotine, alcohol, and a vast range of xenobiotic chemicals that are found in our food and water supply. Women consuming alcohol on a regular basis during pregnancy are more likely to give birth to autistic children.[170] These and other potentially toxic exposures can have more harmful and long-lasting effects on young children than was previously suspected.

The take-home lesson is that we need to be aware of how our children are either developing or not developing, and be perceptive and courageous enough to have them checked out by the appropriate physician if they seem too far removed from their immediate environment—from the people who interact with them. Even though autistic behavior manifests as being out of touch in a profound way, it can often go unrecognized by parents who write it off as "slow development" or a "spacey disposition." Although autism can be difficult to detect very early on, it can be discerned with a high level of accuracy and predictability by the age of eighteen months.[171]

Even with older children, autism can be improved through the methods discussed in this book. That is, largely by adjusting the internal biochemical milieu of a child's brain, it appears possible to greatly augment the behavior of autistic children, regardless of age. Our clinical experience indicates that young autistic children in particular can eventually recover brain function, enabling them to enjoy the full range of social, behavioral, and cognitive activities for which they were genetically endowed.

Chapter 4

◆

Toxic World,
Endangered Mind

Our world turns more toxic with each passing day, yet most of the noxious substances in our environment cannot be experienced in an immediate or palpable sense. We may be alarmed when we see black smoke billowing from a factory or pouring out of a truck's exhaust pipes. We may express disgust at the site of mounds of trash tossed alongside the highway. But we are generally unaware of the minute quantities of mercury vapors we inhale; the traces of pesticides, solvents, and other "permissible" poisons we ingest through our drinking water; or the toxic chemicals in the household objects and cleaners we use on a regular basis.

Our children, of course, are also unaware of these threats to their physical and mental well-being. The trouble is, children are far more vulnerable than adults to the toxic effects of these substances—and fetuses and infants are even more imperiled. As you will see, much of this toxic assault focuses on that most spectacular of evolutionary feats: the human brain.

Each day, thousands of chemicals are being dumped into our air, water, and food supply. Scientists studying the effects of these chemicals say these substances are incurring profound and perhaps irreparable damage to the earth's natural ecosystems. In many cases, this damage may not even become evident until decades later, when genetic anomalies have begun to surface in seagulls and polar bears, or when fish in our oceans, lakes, and rivers begin to develop mysterious epidemics of cancerous tumors.[1] These phenomena among animal populations have alarmed scientists, who worry that similar effects are already occurring in humans. We now know, for example, that toxic effects that occur in one generation can have adverse consequences on brain function and mental health two or even three generations later.

As a practicing physician, I did not trouble myself with these issues for many years. I devoted most of my time and energy to working within the purview of family medicine, which encompasses internal medicine, pediatrics, gynecology, surgery, and preventive medicine. In medical school, we learned very little about the connection between environmental toxins and disease. Most of the education focused instead around diagnosing illness and identifying drugs and other interventions aimed at the elimination of symptoms. In doing so, it seemed clear that we were disregarding the deeper roots of problems that had been developing for months, years, perhaps even decades.

In 1985, my wife died of breast cancer. Until that time, I had believed unequivocally in the power of allopathic (orthodox) medicine—although I had also begun to explore the world of nutritional and preventive medicine. The death of my wife drove home the realization that conventional medical strategies did not always pan out, and that it was often necessary to support the "proven" methods with more innovative strategies. It was time to expand my horizons. My interest in environmental medicine grew out of a desire to learn more about the root causes of illness and to find ways to halt its progress early on, rather than treat it at a stage when it was already far advanced. This new interest also led me also to study nutritional biochemistry, free radical biology, applied immunology, applied toxicology, and environmental and molecular cancer therapy.

Environmental medicine focuses on the impact of the outer world on the fragile ecosystem of the human body—the brain, nervous system, and myriad cellular interactions that must function together in an intricate web of harmonious relationships to ensure good health. Environmental medicine seeks not only to diagnose a person's illness, but to understand its root cause from a holistic perspective, taking into account the complexities of the whole person. Illness is thus understood not only as it shows up in test results or during an examination, but within the context of a person's whole life—living situation, family history, diet, occupation, and history of possible exposure to various toxins and chemicals.

The field of environmental medicine began in the 1950s. At that time it was called *clinical ecology,* a term first used by Theron G. Randolph, M.D., a distinguished allergist who had begun to notice a cause-and-effect relationship between exposure to certain environmental substances (such as chemicals or foods) and allergic-like symptoms in his patients. He was the first physician to recommend labeling prepared food with an exact list of the substances it contained. The publication of Rachel Carson's book *Silent Spring* in 1962 further galvanized the growing field of environmental medicine, drawing a frightening picture of the environmental catastrophes that were occurring in the world.

Other physicians soon picked up on Randolph's environmental approach. William Rea, M.D., a thoracic and cardiovascular surgeon who himself suffered from an environmental illness, led some of the first thorough scientific investigations in this field.

For the environmental medicine specialist, chronic illness is always related in some way to factors in one's environment, and it should not be accepted as something a person just has to live with. This kind of medicine is particularly interested in the potential toxic effects of everyday chemicals around us—and the capacity of this toxic burden to overwhelm all the systems of the body. The toxic burden has the potential to cause long-range debilitating effects that can add up to chronic disease, possibly after years of unwitting exposure to these substances.

My Approach to Environmental Medicine

In my approach, which I call *clinical molecular medicine,* I go even further, integrating environmental medicine with applied immunology, toxicology, and clinical nutritional biochemistry. This allows me to create a comprehensive picture of the role played by these toxic materials. We can then design a multifaceted treatment program that gets to the root causes of a disease. Treatment at our center may include special avoidance diets, nutrition, detoxification (including saunas and chelation therapy), and immunotherapy (e.g., intravenous gamma globulin), among others. All of these regimens are designed to strengthen the body naturally, and help it clear out toxins more effectively.

In my clinical experience, I have found this approach to be particularly effective in treating autism. As I noted earlier, I am convinced that autism is caused by neurotoxic damage, combined with a genetic predisposition for liver dysfunction. It is clear to me that environmental toxins play a central role in the etiology of this disease. The child's body shows a reduced ability to remove heavy metals, probably due to a combination of nutritional deficits and genetic defects in metallothionein, the system that ordinarily helps eliminate these metals. It saddens me to see so many children being treated superficially for this disorder, with therapeutic programs focusing on behavioral modification and education to help them overcome autistic symptoms, when the real cause is within our reach.

I believe treating autism must begin on the molecular level. Only when we have a thorough understanding of the role of toxic substances such as chemicals and heavy metals can we begin to reverse the course of the disease. Again and again, I have seen this pattern in my patients. Autism is intimately linked to the invisible damage that is being done to our children by toxic chemicals that are all around us. This is where we must begin if we are to gain a total picture of this disorder and treat it effectively.

A World Turning Toxic

In a perfect world, all children would have equal opportunities—to be healthy, get a good education, live in a secure environment, and thrive in a carefree world. But the world we live in is far from perfect, as the autism epidemic and other tragic trends make clear. Each day the world grows increasingly unsafe—particularly for our children. Ironically, some of the most profound dangers our families face are the ones the media seemingly downplays or ignores altogether. Crime, automobiles, "stranger danger," and even the Internet can't compare to the single biggest obstacle to our children's ability to thrive: our increasingly polluted environment.

Some 80,000 different chemicals are currently in commerce here in the United States.[2] Many of these chemicals are transmitted into our bodies through the normal food supply. Our daily diet certainly accounts for much of our daily toxic exposures, even though the chemicals only enter us in extremely minute quantities each time we're exposed. More than 2 billion pounds of pesticides are used on our food crops each year. If you're not eating organically grown (pesticide-free) food, chances are you're getting regular doses of these chemicals. Add to that the chemical exposures we routinely receive through our air and water, as well as through medications (both prescription and over-the-counter), personal care and beauty products, dust contaminants (pesticides and heavy metals), cleaning solvents, and household products, and you have a witch's brew of alien and toxic chemicals.

Most of these chemicals or xenobiotics have found their way into the environment over the past five decades, and their numbers are still increasing. The National Institute for Environmental Health Sciences (NIEHS) estimates that more than 2,000 new chemicals are now introduced each year. Here's what the NIEHS has to say about this ever-increasing generation of chemical pollutants: "In 1918, about 10 million pounds of synthetic organic chemicals were produced, used, and disposed of in this country. By 1936, production was up to 860 million pounds a year. The numbers have increased dramatically over the years: 1941, 2 billion; 1944, 37 billion; 1947, 38 billion; 1961, 100 billion; and 1979, 300 billion pounds of synthetic organic chemicals were made, used, and disposed of in the United States. This figure amounts to nearly 1,700 pounds of chemicals for every man, woman, and child in the United States."[3]

How many of the toxic chemicals we produce are actually released into the environment? In 1998, according to the Toxics Release Inventory and other national databases, industries reported releasing 1.2 billion pounds of chemicals into the air and water. This figure is probably a gross underestimate, however, since only 5 percent of the chemicals released into the environment are reported to the national databases.[4] Thus, upwards of 20 billion pounds of chemicals may be released into our air and water each year. Incredibly, over half of these pollutants are known to adversely affect neurodevelopmental functioning.[5]

What are we to make of these mind-boggling numbers? Relatively little is known about the toxicity of many chemicals present in the environment. A number of chemical pollutants are known to damage genetic and cellular structures, causing serious health problems in the process, as I discussed in the preceding chapter. For some children, the chemical exposures translate into an increased risk of developing cancer years or even decades from now. For others, the exposures translate into a much more immediate threat, one that includes autism and other neurodevelopmental deficits. The delicate development of the fetal brain may be the most critical window of vulnerability, as much research now attests.[6]

What We Don't Know Could Be Killing Us

Aside from the relentless burgeoning of this toxic burden, perhaps the most alarming fact is that *most of these synthetic substances have been subjected to little or no research to assess their long-range safety.* We have yet to fully understand their potential impact on younger generations. In 1984, the National Academy of Sciences reported that the U.S. population was likely to be exposed to at least 15,000 of the chemicals registered for commercial use with the EPA. Fewer than half of these chemicals, however, had been evaluated for any toxicity whatsoever, and fewer than one in five had been tested for toxicity in developing lab animals.[7] Moreover, one published study suggests that the tests used to determine chemical toxicity are too insensitive to detect the injury that can potentially result from exposure to these chemicals.[8]

In the preceding section, I alluded to the problem of interactions between different chemicals, even among those that usually exist only at a very low level. We optimistically assume that such *low-level* exposures will not translate into a serious problem. In other words, at sufficiently low doses, most chemicals should be relatively harmless. This may be true, but only *on an individual basis,* depending on specific biological conditions (e.g., immune competence versus immune dysfunction) and the stage of development (later life versus early life). Some chemicals are so powerful that even extremely small doses can have toxic effects—especially on the fragile fetal brain. What's more, in "the real world of multiple and simultaneous exposures," to borrow a phrase from Dr. Marc Lappe in his superb book *Chemical Deception,* even extremely low doses of several chemicals, when presented to the body at the same time, can be quite harmful. In the coming years, we will continue to learn about seemingly innocuous exposures to chemical substances in the air we breathe, the food we eat, and the water we drink and bathe in.

Chemicals classified as toxic are not the only potential threat from chemical pollution. Many of the supposedly "biocompatibile" or nontoxic substances, such as solvents, chemical degreasing agents, and synthetic versions of naturally occurring hormones, have been introduced, only to be recalled or reassessed when adverse effects cropped up. For most of the chemicals of concern, as Dr. Lappe points out, the "science of risk assessment is hamstrung by unknown interactive effects and by only indirectly predictive animal tests. For one thing, risk analysis has yet to devise a way of dealing with the multiplicity of chemical exposures that characterize almost every environmental assault."[9] The combinations of these diverse exposures are extremely difficult, if not impossible, to duplicate in the laboratory.

In short, the pollution burden we now face is far more than the toxins that might first come to mind—the smokestacks of heavy industry and the pesticides used in food production. From the materials in our homes and furnishings to the food we put on our family tables, we routinely encounter hundreds of man-made chemicals that the human body was not designed to ingest or inhale: among them, plastics and petrochemical derivatives, food-borne residues of pesticides and synthetic fertilizers, heavy metals, and many more.

Why Kids are at Special Risk

When other physicians ask me about environmental links with autism, I will often zero in on the indisputable fragility of a child's nervous system in early life. Children today are exposed to thousands of synthetic chemicals, half of which may have neurotoxic properties. These are novel biological experiences: The child is coming in contact with substances never before encountered in our evolution, substances to which the human body cannot adequately adapt. Unfortunately, the developing brains and nervous systems of infants and young children are much more vulnerable to the poisons that surround us in modern life. These facts, taken together, may help explain why a surprising number of U.S. children suffer from neurological disorders such as autism, attention deficit/hyperactivity disorder, dyslexia, and other neurodevelopmental problems—currently about one in every six U.S. children, or approximately 12 million kids.[10]

How do we explain the insidious damage done by environmental toxins to young brains? "More and more we're recognizing that the early stages in the lives of humans and other organisms are particularly sensitive to environmental pollutants," says Richard DiGiulio, a professor of environmental toxicology at Duke University's Nicholas School of the Environment, and director of the new Duke University Superfund Basic Research Center.[11] Children have certain windows of opportunity for developing essential communication skills. If those windows are clouded by damage to the centers of the mind that must learn to perceive, process information from, and develop logically and emotionally appropriate responses to the world, some of those critical skills can be severely, perhaps even irreversibly, compromised.

Why are children, in general, even more vulnerable than their adult counterparts? Philip J. Landrigan M.D., M.Sc., director of the Center for Children's Health and the Environment, offers at least three cogent explanations for children's greater vulnerability to toxins in the environment.[12] The three-point rationale is as follows:

1. **Children have greater exposures to environmental toxins**. There are several reasons for this. First, children tend to absorb pollutants more readily than adults, and retain them in the body for longer periods of time. Second, infants and young children have faster metabolic rates compared to adults. A three-year-old child takes in twice as much air at rest as the average adult on a per-pound body weight basis; also, young children consume three to four times more food when compared to the average adult, again on a per-pound basis.[13] This means that kids are taking in more pollutants from air and food, on a per-pound basis. Dr. Landrigan points out that children further magnify their exposures to toxins in the environment through their hand-to-mouth behaviors and their tendency to play close to the ground; both sets of behaviors tend to boost their exposure to a wide variety of toxins.

2. **Children have weaker detoxifying capacities**. Children have immature metabolic pathways, which means their ability to detoxify and excrete certain toxins differs from that of adults. In most instances, according to Dr. Landrigan, the child's body is less able to deal with toxic chemicals, thus making it more vulnerable to these substances compared to the adult's body. As I've discovered through painstaking research in my Atlanta-based center, autistic children have it even worse: They come into this world genetically predisposed to an even greater degree of vulnerability. Autistic children are hampered in their ability to detoxify because of a seriously defective liver. This predisposes them to massive accumulations of harmful toxins, many of which are neurotoxicants, substances capable of damaging the central nervous system in profound ways.

3. **Toxic chemicals can easily disrupt the development processes that take place within a young child's body**. The nervous, immune, and reproductive systems all undergo rapid growth and development in the first months and years of life. Vital structures within each of these systems are formed during this time and key connections between nerve cells are established. The nervous system actually develops all through childhood (from embryonic development through adolescence); however, this system has minimal ability to repair structural damage caused by toxic pollutants.[14,15] If cells in the young brain are destroyed by chemical pollutants, or if

the critical nerve connections fail to form, there is, according to Dr. Landrigan, a "high risk that the resulting neurobehavioral dysfunction will be permanent and irreversible. The consequences can be loss of intelligence and alteration of normal behavior."[16] To this I would add a key qualifying comment: Many cases are, in fact, reversible as long as the disorder is diagnosed and treated early enough.

Timing is of the essence for a variety of reasons. Over time, many of the chemicals to which our children are exposed can accumulate in the fatty tissues of their bodies, becoming poisons that wreak havoc on delicate cell structures in the brain and elsewhere. In adults, these insults to the sophisticated but fragile chemistry of the body can cause premature aging, higher risks of cancer, and degenerative illnesses, among other woes. In children, we now know, the bodily systems that handle chemicals carry even greater fragility.

We have only begun to glimpse at how deeply vulnerable these younger generations are toward the now-toxic environment we have been polluting. However, the further we trace our lives back to their source, the more vulnerable we become to the assaults of environmental pollution. Many pollutants to which a mother is exposed—such as lead, mercury, and polychlorinated biphenyls (PCBs)—are particularly dangerous to the developing fetus and infant. Both prenatal and postnatal exposures to lead can lead to lifelong cognitive deficits and behavioral disorders.[17] PCBs in the drinking water may be linked with injury to the developing brain in utero,[18] and children exposed to PCBs in the womb had significantly lower IQ scores as well as significant memory and attention deficits.[19] Mercury is a potent and ubiquitous neurotoxicant that can cause severe damage to the developing brain, and the observation that mercury can leach from dental amalgams remains a matter of grave concern.[20,21] Even very low-level exposures to mercury can be harmful to the fetus.[22] This is of special concern, since the EPA recently announced that mercury exposures to the general population appear to be far more common than previously thought.

Equally insidious—and much harder to study—is the damage incurred on both sperm and egg before the embryo even begins to take shape in the mother's womb. I believe this is where the roots of most autistic disorders lie.

Figure 4-1

The Crisis of Early-Life Exposure to Chemical Pollution

There is now reason to believe that prenatal or postnatal exposure to toxic substances play a critical role in over half of all children with autism, learning disabilities, and other developmental impairments. According to the Center for Children's Health and the Environment, affiliated with the Mount Sinai School of Medicine, common pollutants such as lead, mercury, PCBs, and certain pesticides are likely contributors to a substantial fraction of these widespread neurodevelopmental disorders.[23] Unfortunately, as the National Institute of Environmental Health Sciences noted in 1999, research agencies and institutions have only begun to address the environmental hazards confronting our infants and children.[24]

The effects of this toxic soup on children can be devastating. While probably most children can handle mild environmental "insults" to our well-being, those who are exposed to multiple toxins or to higher levels of individual toxins—or who display a compromised ability to process these toxins—are at serious risk for significant problems. The Environmental Protection Agency recently acknowledged that autism may be the result of "neurotoxicants" that interfere with normal developmental processes in the nervous system.[25] My research shows that autistic children clearly lack the biological support to protect their developing bodies from toxic chemicals and heavy metals.

Understanding the Toxic Milieu

Toxic chemicals and heavy metals saturate the environment in which we live, and there is no way to avoid them completely. PCBs have been found in the tissues of every kind of living creature on earth. Lab tests are likely to find an average of about 250 toxic contaminants in a specific individual's body fat, no matter where on the planet he or she lives.[26]

Because the neurotoxic effects of most of these substances have not yet been thoroughly tested, they are found in products and chemicals that we use every day. Many are so ubiquitous that we'd never think twice about using the substances that bring us into contact with them. They are intimately interwoven into our daily lives, and include components of gas, paints, glues, plastics, pesticides, and other common substances.

There are all kinds of poisons lurking in any ordinary household. Because products such as spray cleaners, dishwashing liquids, pesticides, and polishes are legal, we tend to assume that the FDA is protecting us, that these products can't really be hazardous if they are legal. Nothing could be further from the truth. A single exposure to the dangerous chemicals in these products might not be debilitating, but prolonged exposure can lead to all manner of chronic health problems.

For example, aerosols contain isobutane, a compound that doesn't destroy the earth's ozone layer as freon did, but has proven toxic to the heart and central nervous system in laboratory animals. Wood polishes may contain phenol, which has been shown to cause cancer in animals; and residual vapors of these substances can remain in your home long after they are applied. Glass cleaners contain ammonia, which is poisonous when inhaled. Newsprint, mascara, cookware, and piping all contain lead. Automobile exhaust contains mercury, benzene, and carbon monoxide. House and garden pesticides contain synthetic toxic chemicals that have been linked to birth defects, leukemia, and cancer. Mercury vapors given off by dental amalgams enter the mother's bloodstream and are passed on to the developing fetus and, via breast milk, to the breast-feeding child. And the list goes on.

Since the beginning of the industrial revolution we have been pumping millions of tons of chemical substances into the environment. Many of these substances are now turning up in seemingly innocuous places, in our homes and workplaces. Benzene, perhaps the most ubiquitous of all toxic chemicals, has been shown to cause leukemia in workers exposed continuously to it in high concentrations. Benzene is found in gasoline, tobacco smoke, and many common household products. Most people come into contact with this chemical through secondhand smoke or car exhaust, rather than through industrial pollution of the atmosphere. One study showed that people in the United States absorb 45% of their total exposure to benzene from smoking, or breathing in secondhand smoke; 36% from inhaling gasoline fumes or the fumes of glues and other household products; and 16% from other sources in the home. Only 3% of the total exposure came from industrial pollution.[27]

The typical modern home, although widely assumed to be a safe haven from the dangers of the outside world, contains some of the most potent toxins we come into contact with. We breathe in heavy metals through house dust and chloroform in the shower or laundry room as chlorinated water evaporates.[28] Many individuals have toxic reactions to the chemicals emitted by certain carpets, including nervous system dysfunction and difficulty breathing.[29] When ground water—and drinking water—in an area of Tucson, Arizona, was contaminated with tricholorethylene (TCE), a solvent used for cleaning metal, the chemical dramatically increased symptoms of lupus erythematosus in people in the area.[30]

The workplace can be extremely hazardous as well. Workers in certain industries regularly come into contact with toxic organic solvents such as benzene, toluene, kerosene, varnish, and many others. Women whose occupations expose them to these chemicals, such as dry cleaning, lab work, or industrial work, have been shown to have a much higher incidence of major fetal malformations or spontaneous abortions. Organic solvents may also be a cause of multiple sclerosis.[31]

To give you an idea of the magnitude of this problem, here is an overview of the effects of a few of the toxic substances that most of us are unwittingly exposed to every day. I will address their specific effects in greater detail in later chapters.

The Menace of Toxic Metals

Heavy metal poisoning—dangerously high exposure to lead, mercury, cadmium, nickel, and tin, as well as poisoning with other toxic metals such as aluminum and arsenic—is the most widespread environmental illness in the United States today.[32] Exposure to toxic metals is associated with autism, learning and behavioral problems, mental retardation, and other developmental problems. We absorb heavy metals into our bodies through the air, water, and food. Exposure to toxic metals may account for as much as 20 percent of learning disabilities, 20 percent of all strokes and heart attacks, and in some areas be a factor in over 40 percent of birth defects.[33]

Even slight exposure to heavy metals can damage a child's ability to learn. The effect of these toxic metals—aluminum, arsenic, cadmium, lead, tin, and mercury—on a child's mental capacities should not be underestimated. Prenatal and postnatal exposure to these substances is responsible for impairments in these areas, possibly explaining up to 20 percent of cognitive differences among children who have low levels of exposure *not exceeding health guidelines*.[34]

The problem is multilayered, and exacerbated by poor nutrition. Lack of certain key nutrients can render the body even more vulnerable to the toxic effects of heavy metals. These metals may disrupt the balances of certain nutrients in the body, such as calcium levels in cells that affect the release of neurotransmitters, as well as magnesium, lithium, zinc, iron, and vitamins B_6 and B_{12}. Deficiencies in these nutrients, in turn, have actually been shown to increase the neurological damage that heavy metals can inflict.[35,36]

Two of the heavy metals that are most problematic, because of their potency and ubiquity, are mercury and lead.

Mercury. Mercury is a natural element, produced in the breakdown of minerals in rocks and soil from wind, water, and volcanic activity. Over time, the level of mercury to which humans are exposed has been steadily rising. Furthermore, since the beginning of the industrial revolution there has been a continued increase in industrial production through mining and the burning of fossil fuel, which has led to an exponentially higher amount of mercury being released into the atmosphere. The air has three to six times the mercury it did in 1800. The Environmental Protection Agency maintains that this level does not pose a threat to our health; nonetheless, they also have yet to determine what levels in air pollution might be damaging to a fetus via the mother's bloodstream. A presumably acceptable level may in fact be *unacceptable* as mercury levels build up in the body. I cannot help but speculate that mercury exposure in prenatal life is one of the missing links in the massive epidemics of chronic disease humans have faced since the dawn of the industrial revolution.

Perhaps the most widespread and insidious source of mercury exposure today may be dental amalgams, the alloys that compose the "silver" fillings used to repair cavities. The same fillings that fill many an adult American mouth are 50 percent mercury—the second most poisonous substance on earth. Human and animal studies on mercury toxicity, as well as the amount of mercury released from amalgam fillings, suggest that this is a matter of serious concern whose potential dangers have been grossly neglected.[37] This mercury may leach out or vaporize in the mouth and enter a person's bloodstream through the sensitive tissues of the mouth. As I noted earlier, the mercury travels through the pregnant mother's bloodstream and is transferred across the placenta to the fetus.

Following birth, the biggest source of exposure to mercury in infants and young children is the breast milk of a mother who has amalgam fillings.[38] I have encountered cases of infants and children who had significant burdens of mercury and whose mothers had a higher than normal number of amalgams. Many of the parents have evidenced the same levels of mercury exposure as their children; however, it is clearly the latter who suffer most from this exposure. These children suffer from various forms of neurological impairment, ranging from autism to ADHD. Eating fish is another major source of mercury. In this context, too, the mercury can be transmitted from mother to child via breast milk.

In the human body, neurons are among the most vulnerable cells in the body to the neurotoxic effects of methylmercury (a form of organic mercury).[39] In effect, methylmercury kills human neurons. As always, the developing central nervous system of the infant and fetus is highly sensitive to the damaging effects of this toxic metal. Not only does mercury damage nerve cells directly, but it also damages the blood-brain barrier meant to protect the brain from such toxins, and it goes on to generate free radicals that further damage nerve cells. Hundreds of studies have shown the neurotoxic effects of mercury, even at very low doses.[40] In a recent study, prenatal mercury exposure as low as 10 parts per million impeded the brain development of the fetus.[41]

Some of the most common symptoms of mercury toxicity—in both children and adults—are irritability, shyness, tremors, changes in mood and personality, changes in vision or hearing, loss of memory, and loss of sensation or muscle coordination. I will talk more about the direct relationship between mercury toxicity and autism in the next chapter.

Lead. Exposure to lead is widespread through contact with peeling paint in old houses and apartments, as well as older water pipes. This toxic metal is commonly found in household dust, soil, pipe solder, and some ceramics. Though leaded gasoline has been banned in technologically advanced countries, leaded gasoline exhaust still poses a major health problem in many developing countries.[42] Lead poisoning has been linked to infantile autism[43] as well as a whole range of developmental problems, including mental retardation, learning disabilities, attention deficit disorder, and hyperactivity.[44,45] The nature of the damage depends on the timing and extent of the exposure—the brain of the fetus being the most vulnerable.

Despite considerable progress in "getting the lead out" of the United States since the 1970s, nearly 1 million children up to five years of age had higher blood lead levels during the four years they were tested in the 1990s.[46] At low concentrations once deemed to be safe, lead can reduce a child's IQ and promote reading and learning disabilities.[47] (Imagine the extent of damage that might result from relatively heavy lead exposures!) Paradoxically, a recent study found that even quite low levels of lead had a more severe impact on intelligence than was previously believed. Even at concentrations much lower than those deemed unsafe by U.S. government standards, lead can substantially impede a child's ability to learn.[48] In a seven-year study of 309 children in Yugoslavia, lead exposure was most damaging to perceptual-motor skills, rather than language-related aspects of intelligence.[49]

Once again, the windows of greatest vulnerability are fetal life, infancy, and early childhood. Any lead exposure during these time frames can have far-reaching consequences on neurological health in the future. Such damage may go far beyond the problems we usually associate with declining health. Levels of lead in the bone have been linked with antisocial and delinquent behaviors in childhood, and even predicted criminality in adulthood.[50]

I should point out that girls exposed to lead will then store the metal in their bones. Years later, when they become pregnant, this lead will be released, thus exposing their fetuses. A recent study found that many U.S. women of childbearing age still have blood levels considered to be excessive.[51] Like PCBs and other persistent pollutants, lead exposure represents a long-range health hazard, one that is both directly and indirectly passed on to subsequent generations.

In addition to the threat of metals, we have numerous chemical threats to deal with. The two major groups are solvents and pesticides.

The Not-So-Safe Side of Solvents

Hundreds of the chemicals to which we are regularly exposed do not simply pass through the body, but instead accumulate in the adipose (fat) tissues of the body. Since 1976, the EPA has overseen a program that collects and chemically analyzes a nationwide sample of human adipose tissue for the presence of toxic compounds. The agency's purpose is to determine how widely these toxic compounds are distributed in the U.S. population. In 1982, when the EPA expanded its list to include fifty-four different chemical toxins, five chemicals were found in every single one of the samples tested.[52] One of these chemicals was a dioxin; the four others were *solvents*, chemicals used in cleaning agents, paints, cosmetics, and many industrial processes. At various doses, solvents may interfere with the normal development and functioning of the brain and nervous system.[53]

Toluene, used in various cosmetics and a known neurotoxin, was found in approximately 95 percent of the samples tested by the EPA. Women exposed to toluene-containing products prior to, during, or soon after pregnancy may unwittingly pass on the neurotoxic chemicals to the developing fetus. Even in adults, normal psychomotor and cognitive functioning can become impaired by exposure to toluene-containing vapors.[54,55] The neurotoxic effects become greatly amplified in the very young. Keep in mind, also, that the chemical burden in the pregnant or lactating mother will not show up in blood measures, but must be determined by measuring concentrations in body fat. I return to this point in later chapters.

In the industrial setting, workers in a wide variety of jobs—automotive repair, sewage treatment, painting, and construction—are frequently exposed to chemical solvents used for various cleaning purposes. These individuals may suffer neurological and behavioral impairments as a result of their daily exposure to these chemicals.[56,57] For example, sewage treatment workers in New York City experienced frequent fatigue, headache, and light-headedness—symptoms consistent with central nervous system damage resulting from solvent exposure.[58] Spray painters showed poor concentration and other forms of mental dysfunction.[59] Automotive repair shop workers with regular solvent exposures performed poorly on memory and visual perception tests.[60]

In my Atlanta-based center, I routinely measure xylene and styrene in blood. These two neurotoxic solvents were found in 100 percent of the EPA's samples. The excessive accumulation of such solvents in a child's body is a good indicator that his or her liver is not functioning up to par. The accumulation is also likely to be associated with specific nerve-damaging effects.

Other commonly found solvents linked with nerve damage include trichloroethylene (found in dry-cleaning fluid), benzene, trimethylbenzene, N-hexane, methanol, and ethanol (alcohol). Allow me to briefly describe two of the more ubiquitous and dangerous of these solvent compounds: n-hexane and trimethylbenzene.

N-hexane. N-hexane is an industrial solvent used in rubber, glue, paint, lacquer, and printing industries. People involved in certain industries—particularly the shoe industry, in which n-hexane is used as a component of glue—may be exposed daily to dangerously high levels of n-hexane without even knowing it, usually by inhaling it. (Glue sniffers are often exposed to high levels of n-hexane mixed with other solvents.)

N-hexane has been shown to have chronic neurotoxic effects, causing polyneuropathy, as well as severe damage to the central nervous system.[61]

Trimethylbenzene (TMB). Trimethylbenzene is a major component of industrial solvents used in the paint and lacquer industries. We sometimes find elevated levels of this substance in the blood tests of our autistic patients. TMB has been shown to have neurotoxic effects. In one study, short-term inhalation of this compound induced persistent behavioral alterations in rats, which remained evident weeks after exposure.[62]

The Peril of Pesticides

Pesticides have been associated with a host of developmental problems in children, from cognitive deficits to motor skill impairments to aggression and irritability. The frightening thing is there is really no way to completely avoid exposure to pesticides. Drinking water in most states is contaminated with several varieties of pesticide. We thus absorb them not only through the produce we buy at the grocery store that has been sprayed with pesticides, but also through our skin, in the shower, and through rain and drinking water.

Chemicals in pesticides are known to impair learning and motor skills in children. One study of a Yaqui Indian community in Mexico found that children living in a valley where large amounts of agricultural pesticides are used showed significant impairments in gross and fine hand-eye coordination, thirty-minute recall, stamina, and drawing ability.[63] The four- and five-year-old subjects of the study fared substantially worse in such areas than neighboring children of the same age, who live in the nearby foothills where families avoid using agricultural chemicals to control garden pests. The pesticide-exposed children had difficulty drawing even a simple human stick figure, while the foothills children had no trouble completing this task. Farmers in the valley apply pesticides forty-five times per crop cycle, and grow one to two crops per year. So perhaps it is not surprising that children in the Yaqui Valley are born with concentrations of many pesticides in their blood, and are further exposed through breast milk.

Chemicals in pesticides have a host of other harmful effects. One five-year study of the effect of common pesticides on male mice showed damage to the nervous, immune, and endocrine systems.[64] Certain pesticides made the rats more aggressive and irritable. The researchers suggested that this may be because certain pesticides are known to affect thyroid hormone levels, in both rats and humans. The danger of this effect is increased, according to the study's authors, because people receive heavy "pulse" doses of these pesticides when the chemicals are sprayed on crops at certain times of the year. This makes it easier for these toxins to circumvent the body's natural defense systems against them. Such pulse doses of fertilizer could also prove extremely harmful if encountered during some critical window of development early in gestation.

Figure 4-2

Examples of Harmful Chemicals in Our Environment

- *Pesticides:* DDT, 1,4-dichlorobenzine, hexachlorobenzene, transnanochlor.

- *Aromatic organic chemicals (all solvents):* benzene, toluene, xylene, styrene.

- *Chlorinated and brominated organic chemicals:* PCBs, chloroform, tetrachloroethane, 1,2-dichlorobenzne.

- *Recreational drugs:* cocaine, amphetamines, poppers (amyl nitrite), heroin.

- *Toxic heavy metals:* lead, mercury, cadmium, etc.

- *Phenols, phthalates:* ethylphenol, butylbenylphthalate.

As I have said, children are particularly vulnerable to the effects of all of these toxins. They respond very differently from adults to such exposure. For one thing, they're exposed to proportionally larger amounts of toxins, and as they grow and develop, their potential for damage to the developing systems in their bodies is greater than it is for adults. Environmental agents that mimic the activity of hormones pose a special danger to children, since they may interfere with the differentiation and growth of certain tissues in the body.[65] The epidemic of scrotal cancer among puberty-age chimney sweeps of Victorian England are a good example; they were likely exposed to carcinogenic, hormone-interfering soot while the scrotum was undergoing such differentiation.[66]

Proportionally, children are exposed to more food, water, and air than adults are. Because they grow, children eat more than adults, three to four times more per unit of body weight.[67] Infants and children drink more than two and one-half times as much water daily as adults, in relation to their body weight. They breathe closer to the floor, where chemicals that are heavier than air, such as methyl mercury, may be concentrated.[68] They also can be exposed to heavy metals through ordinary house dust, particularly dust that accumulates in carpets. And children take in more oxygen than adults—a resting infant breathes in twice the amount of air as that of an adult under similar conditions.[69]

Fetal exposure to toxins can occur without the mother even knowing it, since it can involve toxins to which she was exposed months or years earlier. A child can be exposed in the womb to toxins that the mother may be carrying in the fatty tissues of her body, from long before conception occurred. PCBs and lead are two toxic substances that are known to be stored in the mother's tissues and then mobilized during pregnancy and transmitted to the fetus.[70] Many chemical compounds, such as carbon monoxide, are now known to cross the placental barrier, which was once thought to protect the fetus from such exposure.

Toxic defects can be transmitted, it seems, not only through the mother's bloodstream, but also through both the ovum and the sperm. The ovum, which is formed during the fetal stage of the mother, reflects the chemical exposures of both the mother and grandmother![71] Studies have also shown that children of not only mothers but also *fathers* employed in occupations that expose them to hazardous chemicals run a greater risk of neurological impairments and other birth defects.[72]

Parents of autistic children often ask me about the kinds of toxins to which they may be inadvertently exposing their children. Because these substances are so ubiquitous in our environment, they are difficult to avoid. We know that the children of industrial workers exposed to solvent vapors appear to be at greater risk than others for autism and other developmental problems. Later in this book I will address the issue of preconceptual prevention, and purification of the home environment for an autistic child.

Endangered by Environmental Estrogens

Some chemical pollutants have the capacity to disrupt the normal production and activities of hormones, the chemical messengers that help regulate vital body systems. Many of these hormone disruptors are called *xenoestrogens,* because they have estrogen-like activity. A recently published book, *Our Stolen Future,* depicts this phenomenon in stark detail, showing how synthetic chemicals that mimic human estrogen, such as PCBs and pesticides like DDT, have insinuated their way into the tissues and cells of every living being on the planet. These chemicals are causing birth defects and reproductive problems in offspring within animal populations worldwide, from herring gulls in Lake Ontario to sheep in western Australia. These findings have dramatic ramifications for our understanding of these chemicals' effects on humans, and may help explain phenomena such as declining sperm counts worldwide.

Because environmental science has tended to focus on chemicals that cause cancer, there has until recently been little attention paid to this connection between such chemical exposure and epidemics of infertility and sexual dysfunction among the offspring of exposed animals. Similar connections are beginning to crop up in human populations, although this area of research is rife with controversy.

In May 1996, a panel of international experts called for an investigation of a number of hormone-disrupting chemicals that threaten brain and nervous system development. This call came in the wake of a 1991 gathering of experts in Italy, in which scientists had emphasized the sensitivity of the developing brain to chemical damage, which could show up later in the form of reduced intelligence, learning disabilities, and attention deficit problems.[73]

A paper published later that same year, in September 1996 in the *New England Journal of Medicine,* confirmed these findings. The study showed that higher than normal levels of PCBs in the blood and milk of the mothers of 212 children were directly correlated with the children's deficits in intellectual ability, short- and long-term memory, and focused and sustained attention.[74] Similar deficits had been found in these same children as infants. In an earlier study, the infants had exhibited impaired motor coordination, short-term memory, and verbal skills. When the children were eleven years old, the impairments were found to be persistent and significant. Neither a good education nor a supportive environment had been able to compensate for these impairments.[75]

I find this study instructive for several reasons. First, PCBs were once widely used in electric transformers, paper recycling, and other commercial processes. Although their use has been discontinued, the compounds are so stable and persistent that they remain widespread in the environment. Second, being fat soluble, they become concentrated in animal products and in the people that eat those products. Third, we know that nursing mothers can transfer their own internal supply of PCBs to their infants through breast milk or, earlier, to the developing fetus.[76] Many environmental estrogens and other fat-soluble chemicals may follow a similar pattern.

Researchers theorize that exposure to environmental estrogens at various stages of gestation interferes with the fragile and rapidly organ systems in the fetus. The nature and extent of the damage often depends on the time of exposure. Aside from the effects on reproductive health I mentioned earlier, widespread dissemination of environmental estrogens has been linked with congenital malformations (recall the birth defects linked with DES and thalidomide, both considered synthetic estrogens) and neurobehavioral dysfunction in early childhood.[77] There is a thalidomide link to autism as well. Exposure to these hormone disruptors during pregnancy may have a substantial negative impact on long-range health because of the particular vulnerability of developing organ systems. Such hormone-related disturbances in early development can lead to lifelong changes in behavior.[78]

A Lifetime of Toxic Insult

My clinical experience has taught me that chronic disease—including autism and other developmental disorders—is not simply the direct result of exposure to toxins, either prenatally or postnatally. The process is more complex than that. A toxic event in the brain may occur at a certain point in time, but once this injury has occurred, subsequently a host of other symptoms—with different labels, not appearing to be directly related to the toxic event—may appear.[79]

Diseases triggered by exposure to toxins are often hard to spot. One reason is that toxic chemicals tend to target the body's communication systems, such as the nervous system, immune system, and endocrine system, rather than specific organs in the body.[80] This makes the body particularly vulnerable to future exposures, since these are the very systems that are meant to protect us from toxic harm, particularly the immune system. When they're not functioning properly, it makes us even more vulnerable to toxic exposure. And the chemical exposure event may trigger a multi-disease, multistage process, in which a multitude of symptoms may appear months or years after the exposure occurs—making it even harder to pinpoint the original cause of the disease. Genetic defects may take years to manifest.

I would say there are three reasons that some children suffer learning disabilities and other neurological problems while others do not—genetics, nutrition, and environmental toxins. We cannot say much about the genetic aspect, except that we have observed that there can be a genetic "predisposition" to immune or liver detoxication abnormalities leading to allergic sensitivities or toxic overload, which in turn trigger problems such as neurological and cognitive impairment. For example, if a three-year-old child has a particular genetic enzyme defect, he or she may need six times the normal amount of vitamin B_6 to accomplish the same neurochemical processes as a normal child. This affected child may develop a significant learning disability because of this lack of vitamin B_6, even though the parent may be giving him a vitamin supplement with some B_6 in it.

Because of biochemical individuality—each human body's unique response to similar groups of chemical substances—the nutritional aspects of chronic diseases, learning disabilities, and neurological problems are quite diffuse and complex. Our food supply has been corrupted by the food industry, starting with the farm site and carrying right through to the factories that process the foods. The farmer does not grow organic foods, so chemicals contaminate the food. The farmer uses soil over and over, depleting the minerals in it. The food-manufacturing plants process the food so it will have a long shelf life. All of this did not happen in 1790. Thanks to all these processing techniques, foods have lost a large percentage of their nutrient value. What happens as a result of the farmer's and food processor's techniques is that we eat a product that is alien to our systems. A poor food supply leads to poor fuel for the neurochemical processes necessary for learning. Food which lacks appropriate nutrients—thanks to poor farming techniques and processing for long shelf life—in essence starves a child's brain of what it needs to function properly. These nutrient deficiencies can result in learning disabilities.

Finally, there is the immediate environmental impact on the human nervous system. It has been said that the air in our world today has 30 percent less oxygen in it than the world in which prehistoric man lived. Might this have some impact on our health and nervous systems? This, of course, is in addition to the trillions of tons of chemicals and heavy metals we put in our bodies through the air, water, and food supply. If nothing else, this situation certainly has a damaging impact on our molecular systems.

Children have the added disadvantage that they can't remove themselves from a potentially toxic environment. We place our children in classrooms for six hours a day, five days a week. In those thirty hours they breathe in chemicals from carpets, paints, pesticides, toxic cleaning fluids, furniture, office machinery, etc. Schools are often built, for economic reasons, on undesirable land—near a freeway, for example. In addition, most schools are contaminated with molds, to add another major burden to the child who is not adapting well to his environment. And if the school building is more than twenty-five years old, you can add in the asbestos factor. Therefore, alien chemicals, heavy metals, and contaminated air and water can cause an individual child's immune system to become damaged. This can cause sensitivities to certain foods, chemicals, preservatives, and molds. As a result, the child may develop learning disabilities or other problems.

The key to such problems, however, is not only the degree of toxic insult, but also how efficiently the liver rids the body of these toxins. Every chronic disease patient I have treated suffers from detoxication problems as well as a genetic predisposition to develop the disease. If the two phases of liver detoxication are out of balance with each other, the liver is unable to effectively remove toxins that enter the body, and may in fact contribute to the generation of more toxins. These conditions are aggravated by poor nutrition, which depletes the liver of substances required to eliminate toxic chemicals. (Note: This does not apply to heavy metals, which must be removed by natural chelators such as lipoic acid, NAC, glutathione, and cysteine.)

As we have seen, toxic chemicals also disrupt immune function. Accumulation of toxic chemicals and heavy metals in the body may reduce immune function to as little as 50 percent of its original capacity.[81] The immune system may become either suppressed or hyperactivated, resulting in allergies or autoimmune disorders. The hyperactivated immune system triggers a surge in inflammation and free radicals. This, in turn, leads to DNA injury, as well as damage to cells' mitochondria, which leads to oxidative damage resulting in chronic illnesses such as arthritis, chronic fatigue, and central nervous system degenerative processes.

People build up chemicals in their body fat so that by the time they are in their forties or fifties, most people have accumulated all the toxins they will need to generate disease. Many do come down with some chronic degenerative disease. These chemicals then generate *charged particles called free radicals,* which further damage the brain, nervous system, tissues, and organ systems in the body. The blood-brain barrier does not protect us against free radicals and many chemicals.

For reasons we are now only beginning to understand, autistic children manifest the effects of environmental pollutants early in life. This may be related to damage to the developing nervous system of the fetus, due to exposure to toxins via the mother or in the first few months of life. We are still unraveling the causes of autism, but I believe I have identified the nature of this neurotoxic damage, and the key molecular mechanisms underlying this disease.

What Is Clinical Molecular Medicine?

At the Edelson Center, we practice *clinical molecular medicine*. This approach begins with finding out all the details concerning the fundamental mechanism of a patient's illness. Then we develop molecular techniques to treat and prevent disease. In essence, we find out why a patient is ill, instead of just diagnosing the illness.

This is a totally new approach to treating chronic illness, one that integrates environmental medicine, applied immunology (the study of immune system function), applied toxicology (the study of toxic links with illness), and clinical nutritional biochemistry, a highly sophisticated approach to understanding our nutritional and metabolic needs.

What is unique about our program is that we focus on finding out all the details concerning the fundamental mechanism of a person's chronic illness. We then go about treating the disease, not at the external level where symptoms are manifested, but on the molecular level where problems first arise. We develop molecular approaches to treat and prevent disease.

The word *molecular* is very important here. This means that we go to the basic processes inside the cells that are not functioning properly, in order to find and treat illness. While traditional allopathic medicine tends to treat symptoms of disease, when those symptoms are already full-blown, we instead treat illness during the early dysfunctional period in which toxins and deficiencies are leading to malfunction in the body's cells. Obviously, the patient has symptoms at this time as well. However, we address the underlying causes of these symptoms and attempt to "heal" the body by removing the deeper roots of the illness.

How do we accomplish this? The first step is to learn everything about the patient's life, from birth to the present. This is called a comprehensive environmental history, and takes between sixty and ninety minutes to complete. Then we do a thorough physical examination. Once we have this information, we put together a comprehensive profile of laboratory and other tests that will fill in the "pieces of the puzzle" of the patient's illness.

Only then can we explain why people become ill, and how we can help them heal their bodies. The human organism can heal itself if the impediments to the healing process are removed and the body is given the proper nutrients to function efficiently. Our healing program involves the following techniques:

(1) *Biodetoxification*—removing heavy metals and chemicals from the body.

(2) *Nutritional therapy*—oral and intravenous vitamins, minerals, amino acids, and other important nutrients.

(3) *Immunotherapy*—using various natural therapies to help normalize a dysregulated immune system.

(4) *Desensitization*—building resistance into the immune system so that allergies and sensitivities can be eliminated.

(5) *Antibiotic therapy*—natural or traditional therapies to rid the body of unwanted invaders (viruses, bacteria, and fungi).

This is a totally different approach from the long-standing, generally accepted medical tradition of treatment of chronic disease, which has been to attempt to identify the illness by name and then treat the symptoms. In that orthodox medical approach, there is never an attempt to identify the basic cause of the illness and heal the body. It is just not part of the medical school curriculum to teach how to find the molecular roots of the illness. This traditional type of treatment often does more harm than good, since drugs can severely damage the body. There is a growing trend in medicine today to investigate other approaches, focusing on the immune system, nutrition, prevention, and the molecular characteristics of disease. This is where our philosophy lies.

Since I saw my first autistic patient in 1994, I have found this approach to be highly effective in treating children with autism. In these young patients, the behavioral symptoms of autism are only the tip of the iceberg. They reflect a complex process of disease, triggered by toxic exposure and exacerbated by liver dysfunction and poor nutrition. Without understanding and addressing all aspects of this illness, we would be merely applying "Band-aids" to solve behavioral problems. Our approach goes far deeper, identifying and addressing the molecular causes of the disease. We treat the whole person, not merely the symptoms. In this way, we achieve much more substantial and lasting results.

Maggie's Story

Maggie was cherished and adored from the moment she entered the world—her doting parents' first child and the joy of their lives. The pretty, delicate infant with big brown eyes grew into a cherubic toddler, who by her second birthday spoke few words but intrigued those around her with her pleasant, peaceful demeanor.

Then, gradually, inexorably, a darker reality began to emerge. In the year that followed, Maggie's parents knew something was very wrong with their child. Instead of engaging with the world around her, she withdrew. Her only vocalizations were screaming tantrums. She would not—or apparently could not—make eye contact with her parents. She contorted her tiny body into bizarre postures and would rock her body and roll her head back and forth for hours at a time.

Maggie was diagnosed with classic autism, and the prognosis was not good. Conventional medicine attempts to manage, rather than actually treat, autism by using behavioral therapy and drugs to at least stabilize— and hopefully retrain—the autistic behavior. For Maggie, however, such efforts were clearly not fruitful. In response, she seemed to withdraw even further into the mysterious shell of isolation that was hardening around her. But her parents refused to give up hope.

When Maggie was brought to me, she had already seen no fewer than twenty medical doctors for her condition. Her parents were understandably exhausted. "Please help us," Maggie's mother pleaded. "We just want our beautiful baby back."

I ran an exhaustive battery of tests on her, looking for telltale signs of toxic poisoning and biochemical aberrations. Over the years, as I had seen other children like Maggie. I had become more interested in how a genetic predisposition—either hereditary or genotoxic (resulting from damage to the parents' germ cells)—could be triggered by environmental factors to produce autism. The more I looked, the more I found—until I had amassed a unique body of data that supported this thesis. In Maggie's case, I did not have to look hard.

The first set of laboratory studies focused on her blood, which showed elevated levels of xenobiotic substances. Her major problem consisted of mercury toxicity, first and foremost, followed by an array of chemical pollutants that tend to stay lodged in the body's fatty tissues. We found an array of hydrocarbons including hexane, pentane, xylene, benzene, and trimethylbenzene. Among the more common sources of these chemicals are pesticides, herbicides, detergents, cleaning solvents, plastics, and various pharmaceuticals. The blood levels of these fat-soluble chemicals are, on average, only about one hundredth of the levels found in body fat. In addition to the mercury, we found unusually high levels of other heavy metals that are notoriously toxic to developing nervous systems.

All told, Maggie presented me with an astonishing picture of toxicity. Just as ominously, her blood panels showed the effects of a chronic lack of certain key nutrients, including numerous vitamins and minerals that the body needs to sustain normal functioning. She had multiple allergies, manifesting as abdominal pain, runny nose, and watery eyes. We have found that every autistic child has some form of allergy, but in Maggie's case the die seemed even more loaded. I interviewed her parents exhaustively and learned that there were many aspects of their home that may have further added to this picture of burdened immunity, such as chemical cleaning products, new paint, and pesticides.

Our integrated treatment of Maggie, like our treatment for most other children with this disorder, focused primarily on the following measures: nutritional supplementation, detoxification (sauna to remove chemicals, and chelation to remove heavy metals); healing of her digestive system; use of digestive enzymes; behavior modification; and reduction of her allergies by using an avoidance diet. Several of the supplements Maggie took were designed to redress imbalances in her liver's functioning; other supplements were aimed at improving brain function and protecting the brain cells from further injury while her liver function improved.

Today, to everyone's amazement, Maggie is a happy, healthy, vibrant girl. She talks, laughs, and plays with other children. She attends a mainstream prep school and is doing as well as her peers. She is just one of dozens of children I have helped.

Let's Face Facts

Modern science doesn't know why increasing numbers of children are withdrawing into the mysterious world of autism. But it is hard to ignore the data I have compiled showing exceedingly high levels of toxins in their blood and tissues. It is hard to ignore the data showing a rapid recovery process after removing the toxins using a variety of measures. Taken together, these data can lead to only one conclusion: Toxic substances are wreaking havoc on the emotional and cognitive capacities of babies and young children.

As I documented in Chapter 1, autistic kids evidently lack the capacity to handle the growing burden of toxins imposed by the modern environment. This weakness primarily concerns various forms of liver dysfunction; it may also entail defects in natural chelation ability, either genetically or nutritionally (much research remains to be done to clarify this latter aspect). Like the tiny yellow birds once routinely brought down into coal mines to warn the mine workers of danger, they are truly "canaries in the coal mine," warning us of a world out of balance, a world whose vulnerabilities are quickly seen in its most fragile and precious occupants.

A growing number of studies are also suggesting that America's tainted food and water supplies are contributing to the rising tide of autistic spectrum disorders. As I discussed in the preceding chapter, there is good reason to posit that the clustering of autistic cases in the working-class region of Brick Township, New Jersey, is related to the high levels of toxins that have been documented in the drinking water. Also intriguing are reports that babies exposed prenatally to thalidomide had a greater risk of developing autism.

Chapter 5

◆

Understanding the Autism Complex

My clinical experience with the evaluation and treatment of autistic children has convinced me that autism is not merely a neurological illness, but a complex, multiorgan disease. Autistic behavior is the result of a vicious cycle of toxicity, impaired detoxication, immune dysregulation, and malabsorption of essential nutrients. Autism affects not only the brain and nervous system, but virtually every organ in the body.

In this chapter we will look at the elements of this complex syndrome and how they influence each other, giving rise to a cycle of toxic injury that eventually manifests as autistic behavior. First, let me give you some idea of how I developed this theory.

My interest in the role of environmental factors in autism was sparked in the fall of 1994, during a standard medical evaluation of an autistic boy named Rich. Rich's parents had brought him to me because they believed I could help him with his allergies. They had no reason to believe that I would try to help them figure out *why* he was autistic in the first place. This was the first autistic child I really had a chance to work with. It was then that I began to put together the pieces for an innovative protocol for managing this unique and enigmatic illness.

At that time I had read about Bernard Rimland's work on nutritional biochemistry in autistic children. Rimland had evaluated 4,000 questionnaires filled out by parents of autistic children. Out of those questionnaires, he noted that 318 parents had tried using high-dose vitamin B_6 and magnesium, based on some early research suggesting a therapeutic benefit for autistic children.[1] At least 280 of these parents reported behavioral improvements in response to the supplements. Then I heard a lecture in which Dr. Rimland described how most of his autistic patients have allergies. This observation alerted me to the connection between the immune system and autism.

I began to think about the biological profile of autistic children. Here was a group of children with a brain pathology who also had immune dysregulation. In such a scenario, it was easy to see that an activated immune system could trigger allergies. Could toxins be involved in this process? I wondered. Because of my interest in environmental medicine, I was very attuned to such a possibility. I thought, what would be related to 100 percent of these children having allergies of some sort, and also having injury to the brain? What came to mind, of course, is that there are toxins that will damage both the immune system and the brain and give you both of those patterns.

Lab tests showed that Rich had severe food allergies, overgrowth of yeast and parasites in the gastrointestinal tract, low levels of certain key neurotransmitters, elevation of lipid peroxide which indicated free radical stress, pathological detoxication in the liver, an autoimmune process against myelin, and an activated immune system. Also, his antibody tests showed that he was sensitive to formaldehyde and toluene. His intestinal permeability study revealed a leaky gut. He had low levels of the antioxidant glutathione. At that time, we used an indirect measure of chemical toxicity, which he clearly manifested.

Rich did not undergo much therapy with me, except for nutritional therapy and EPD therapy for his allergies. His symptoms, including his autistic behavior, slowly began to improve. At that time Rich was also receiving various other therapies, including applied behavior analysis.

Soon I began to see other autistic patients. I read *The Biology of the Autistic Syndromes* by Christopher Gillberg and Mary Coleman, which gave me further insight into the complexity of this disease. The more autistic children I treated, the more I became convinced that environmental toxicity played a key role in the etiology of this illness. I decided to perform studies to explore the relationships between environmental factors and autism.

I already knew that autism was associated with environmental factors. In 1975, studies by the NIH showed an increased incidence of chemical occupational exposure in the mothers of autistic children. This had caught my "environmentally trained" eye. Then, I heard that autism reached its highest incidence in heavily industrialized areas. And I knew that a number of environmental chemicals cause neurotoxicity. The more immature the brain, the greater the likelihood of this type of damage. I remembered that Waring in England had found that greater than 90 percent of autistic children do not detoxify normally, due to inadequate phenosulfotransferase activity (an enzyme which helps the liver detoxify foreign chemicals). All of this information fit into the picture of autism as a toxic syndrome that was beginning to take shape.

Initially I decided to prepare what I thought to be a reasonable evaluation for autistic patients, covering all the various factors that might play a role in the pathology of this illness. We tested for nutritional biochemistry characteristics by examining the amino acid analysis and mineral analysis. At that time, we also examined levels of vitamins and essential fatty acids in the body. We tested for liver detoxication, as well as levels of toxic chemicals and toxic metals, immune system characteristics, vaccine antibody characteristics, gastrointestinal function, and intestinal permeability.

After I had prepared this protocol, I presented my own hypothesis: Toxins in genetically predisposed individuals lead to damage to the immune system and activation which leads to various symptoms, as well as toxic injury to the central nervous system, leading to the autistic spectrum. Additionally, the toxic state could lead to intestinal permeability problems with either malabsorption or leaky gut; it could also originate from an overgrowth of organisms, or food allergies that lead to inflammation in the gastrointestinal tract. Clearly there was a highly convoluted and complex process at work in the etiology of autism.

I presented this protocol, along with my theory, to several autism research and support groups in Atlanta. We received donations from laboratories to pay for some of our testing. We began our study of autistic patients, using the evaluation we had developed.

As I treated more autistic patients, I began to see a specific pattern. Tests showed that the liver was abnormal in all the patients. This was the genetic defect we had been looking for. We had discovered both a genetic link and environmental factors at work in this illness. This discovery formed the basis of my theory that the autistic spectrum includes a multiplicity of organic injury in the body.

These experiences led to our formal study of about thirty autistic patients, in order to look at all of the potential immunotoxicological, nutritional, biochemical, gastrointestinal, and detoxication characteristics of these children. (In Chapter 1, I described this study in more detail.) Various laboratories helped support this research. We were looking at a broad spectrum of characteristics in these children.

Let me review for you the results of that initial study. We found that every one of these children suffered from some form of immune dysregulation—low natural killer (NK) cell activity, elevated T cell (CD4/CD8) ratios, myelin basic protein abnormalities. There was something definitely abnormal about every one of the children's immune systems.

We also found that every one of these children suffered from a fundamental form of liver dysfunction. Simply put, instead of getting rid of toxins, the liver dysfunction caused a buildup of toxins. Eight out of every ten of these children (80%) were classic cases of *pathological detoxifiers,* a phrase coined by biochemist Jeffrey Bland. Pathological detoxifiers show a fundamental imbalance between the two phases of liver detoxication—excessive phase I activity, together with a lack of phase II activity.[2] This group of children showed extremely high phase I levels—much higher than I had seen in the average adult population—and phase II was consistently low. The imbalance between these phases has the effect of making the body more toxic over time. With the excess in phase I activity, free radicals and other toxic metabolites rapidly accumulate. With the lack of phase II, the liver is unable to flush out the toxins it generates.

We also found elevated levels of toxic chemicals in almost every child, and in a high percentage of these children we found elevated levels of heavy metals. The three heavy metals we usually found were mercury, tin, and lead, which is very interesting since all three of those are neurotoxins. The types of chemicals that we found were those common in daily life— hexane, the pentanes, and the aromatic hydrocarbons—benzene, trichloro-benzene, trichloromethane. Occasionally we also found organophosphates, pesticides, and chlorinated hydrocarbons.

We looked at this as a total picture, and found there were certain characteristics present in 100% of the children: Their liver detoxication was abnormal, and they were all toxic. So we decided we would try to publish a paper looking at those issues.

In smaller percentages of these children, we found all sorts of systemic manifestations of a toxic situation: 50% had maldigestion, 50% had malabsorption, 80% had zinc deficiencies, 60% had magnesium deficiencies, and approximately 30% had candida overgrowth in their gastrointestinal tracts.

The basic premise I felt I had to get across to the public was that this was both a genetic and an environmental illness. Both pieces of that puzzle had to be there for these children to become autistic. We published a paper in December 1998 in the *Journal of Toxicology & Industrial Health,* showing the abnormal liver detoxication and presence of toxic chemicals in these autistic children. We subsequently studied more than seventy autistic children, and found that 100 percent had abnormal liver detoxication, 100 percent had high levels of toxic chemicals, and a large percent showed high levels of heavy metals.

In recent years, the theory that this is mainly a genetically determined disease has gained widespread acceptance. Dr. Nancy Minshew, of the Western Psychiatric Institute and Clinic, an expert in the biology of autism, stated in the April 1996 issue of the *Journal of Autism and Developmental Disorders* that autism is a disorder of neuronal organization caused by severe pathophysiological abnormalities. She doesn't mention why this happens, although it is suggested that it is all due to a genetic defect.

My work shows, however, that autism is not just genetic; it's also toxic. The genetically predisposed infant is like a loaded gun. It takes a toxic environment, however, to pull the trigger.

I never cease to be amazed by how intricately interconnected all our body systems are. Every synapse, neurotransmitter, and metabolic process has to work properly for the body to be in balance and in good health. In an autistic individual, these coordinated processes get thrown out of balance, creating a cycle of toxicity and impaired liver detoxication.

There is a fair amount of agreement in the environmental medicine community that autistic children exhibit certain patterns of abnormalities. Current research on autism seems to focus on these individual phenomena. We have studies of organic acids and their relationship to candida, peptides and their effect on the brain, measles virus in the GI tracts of autistic children, and presence of the stealth virus (a "hidden" virus able to induce disease without causing an inflammatory response) in the brains of some autistic children.[3] But why do these things occur?

Autism as an Immunotoxic Syndrome

None of these findings is difficult to believe when we consider them in light of the fact that these children are *immunotoxic*. Since the late 1980s, it has been known that these children have deficient natural killer (NK) cell activity,[4] which in turn affects their resistance to infection and probably cancer as well. If we give these children vaccines, for example, their bodies are not going to be able to kill off these viruses. Fragmented research in these individual areas is missing the root cause of this problem: These children are toxic, their immune systems are not functioning well, and their livers do not detoxify normally. This is what we need to focus on now.

, I am not suggesting that we should not deal with the specific abnormalities associated with autism. But if we look at only the individual pieces of the puzzle, and forget that *the underlying cause of this process is toxic injury,* we are not going to be able to help these children to improve.

My work with autistic children has shown me that various aspects of compromised immunity, especially weaknesses in NK cell activity, are linked with a host of secondary problems. But what causes this immune deficiency? The answer, again, seems abundantly clear: toxic overload.

The connection between the immune system and autism has been well documented.[5] (I touched on a few of these factors earlier, in Chapter 3.) Immune system abnormalities in autistic individuals have been exhibited as changes in the function of NK cells and T cells, decreased proliferative response to mitogens (substances that stimulate the immune cells), the presence of antibodies to myelin basic protein (myelin is the protective coating surrounding the nerve fibers), and various imbalances involving cytokines, the messengers of the immune system. Until now, these factors have been observed in autistic children, but the relationship between them and autism has not been elucidated.

Let us take a brief look at the evidence for these mechanisms in autistic children. In 1977, Stubbs and colleagues conducted a study of twelve children with autism using mitogen stimulation techniques and concluded that there was a relative T-cell deficiency in autistic children. This deficiency is also seen in toxic chemical and heavy metal burdens. Warren and colleagues studied thirty-one patients with autism and found several immune system abnormalities in the blood. They found, as did Stubbs, that these autistic children had a defective T-cell mitogen response.

In another study, Weizman and colleagues, in 1982, studied cell-mediated immune response to human myelin basic protein by the macrophage inhibition factor test. They compared the results in seventeen patients with autism with those in a control group of eleven patients with other mental conditions. Thirteen of the seventeen patients with autism demonstrated inhibition of migration, while none of the controls did the same. This study suggests that there may be a cell-mediated immune response to brain tissue.

Such changes are observed when toxins affect the human immune system. The question then becomes, what is causing these changes in the status of the immune system in autistic individuals? I would like to suggest that it is no accident that autism—and the immune characteristics associated with it—is increasing in frequency as levels of environmental toxins increase. It is clear to me that the origin of this illness lies in the negative environmental influences on the development of the molecular structures of the brain and the immune system.

A growing body of evidence now suggests autism is not merely an immune disorder, but a disorder with autoimmune characteristics. In 1971, Money and colleagues first raised the possibility that autoimmunity to the brain might play a role in this disorder. One of the clues linking autoimmunity with this problem is high rates of autoimmune disorders exist among families of autistic children. The most common of these disorders, according to Dr. Anne Comi of Johns Hopkins Hospital, include rheumatoid arthritis, type I diabetes, hypothyroidism, and systemic lupus erythematosus. Dr. Comi and her colleagues in the Department of Pediatric Neurology found that these and other autoimmune disorders were eight times more common in mothers with autistic children than in the control group, and five times more common among first-degree relatives of these children compared to relatives of healthy children.[6] More recently, Dr. Comi reported a ninefold increase in the incidence of autism in children born to mothers with autoimmune illnesses.[7]

One of the earliest studies on the autoimmune process in autism, published in 1988, describes antibrain antibodies in autistic individuals.[8] Later studies found significant increases in these abnormal antibodies (called *autoantibodies*) to various brain components (neuronal and glial filament proteins) in autistic children compared to normal children.[9] In children classified within the autistic spectrum (Landau-Kleffner syndrome variant), researchers have found higher levels of serum autoantibodies to brain tissues compared to healthy children.[10] It is now believed that autoimmune damage to the myelin sheath that surrounds nerve fibers may fuel the development of this particular disorder.[11] In my fourth study of autistic children (see Chapter 1), I too found autoantibodies to myelin basic protein and other central nervous system components.

Even laboratory research has begun to support the idea that autoimmunity against key components of the brain and central nervous system may be linked with autistic behavioral symptoms. For example, studies of laboratory rats indicate that autoimmune processes may create a certain behavioral syndrome that could be the animal equivalent of autism.[12] It is now thought that autoimmune mechanisms may contribute not only to autism, but other neurodevelopmental disorders as well.[13]

In April 2001, at the International Medical Conference on Autism in Quebec City, researchers proposed that autism is not merely a neurological disorder, but a systemic illness that involves immunological, gastrointestinal, endocrinological, psychological, and neurological complications.[14] Evidence presented at the conference confirmed the findings in our Atlanta center, as I presented in Chapter 1. These data indicate that some aspects of autism are most likely triggered by a toxic insult to the developing immune system of a fetus, infant, or very young child, which causes the immune system to act against the brain.

In my own clinical practice, as reported in Chapter 1, approximately half of the autistic children I have treated exhibit evidence of an autoimmune process that attacks the brain. This autoimmunity is the result of toxic injury to the fetus or infant in early life.

Manifestations of Immune Imbalance

The types of autoimmune processes that are found in these children often point directly to early toxic injury as the culprit. An imbalance of cytokines, the chemical messengers that direct immune activities, is clearly involved. Broadly speaking, a healthy immune response involves a balance of Th1 and Th2 cytokines. Imbalances of these two groups of cytokines—with a preponderance of the Th2 cytokines linked with allergies and autoimmune disease—may play a role in the development of autism.[15] The Th1 and Th2 shift in cytokines appears to be a critical part of the autoimmune process, observed in both lupus and Graves' disease.[16] The authors of the article suggest that this change in cytokine characteristic is part of the autoimmune pathogenesis of autism—but they note that the precise mechanism for this shift is unknown.

Research has shown, however, that this Th1 and Th2 shift can be caused by mercury, lead, and other environmental pollutants such as trichloroethylene (described below).[17,18] In studies of laboratory animals, the appearance and magnitude of this Th1-Th2 imbalance as well as cellular features of autoimmunity correlated with the dose of mercury administered.[19] Based on this research, it is tempting to speculate that chelation (to remove toxic metals) and other detoxifying strategies could help restore a normal Th1-Th2 balance, perhaps improving the treatment of autism.

Another study, published in 1990, describes a deficiency of a certain class of T helper cells in autism.[20] This particular form of immune deficiency can promote a Th1-Th2 imbalance and the production of antibodies associated with autoimmunity. The researchers found changes in various T-cell subsets—changes virtually identical to those found in autoimmune disorders such as lupus and multiple sclerosis.

It is well known that certain chemicals can accelerate the autoimmune response. One study describes T-cell activation in mice.[21] In the study, mice were exposed through their drinking water to trichloroethylene, an environmental toxin associated with autoimmunity. In the mice, this chemical accelerated an autoimmune response, in association with non-specific activation of Th1 cells. The researchers also found that exposure to trichloroethylene dramatically increased expression of the activation marker CD44 on certain T cells.

This is very significant information, since an increase in the CD44 receptors on T cells points to a further possible autoimmune response. In the same study, an increase in antinuclear antibodies, or ANA, was also observed—another sign of immune dysregulation and autoimmunity. All of this suggests that trichloroethylene—one of many toxic chemicals found in our environment—stimulates or exacerbates an autoimmune response.

Parents of my young patients sometimes ask about the relevance of gamma globulin treatment, and indeed this autoimmune connection may have therapeutic value. Intravenous gamma globulin has been used with good results in some cases.[22] With the immune system abnormalities indicating an autoimmune process, gamma globulin therapy should be effective since it has proven effective in the treatment of many other autoimmune diseases, including chronic inflammatory demyelinating polyneuropathy and multiple sclerosis.

Getting Blood to the Brain: The Coagulation Connection

It is worth mentioning another possible mechanism that may be at work here. This alternative theory has generated a great deal of recent interest because it may help explain the mechanism behind a host of chronic diseases, including autism.

Some studies have shown that autistic patients have reduced blood flow (hypoperfusion) in certain areas of the brain. In one recent study, PET scans revealed decreased blood flow to both sides of the brain (bitemporal hypoperfusion) in autistic people.[23] This phenomenon occurred in regions of the brain that are normally activated by complex speech-like sounds containing spectral modulation (SM). In autistic individuals, there was greater activation of this region on the right side of the brain, while in normal people there was greater activation on the left side. The researchers speculate that perhaps there is an abnormal right shift of auditory processing of speech-like stimuli in autism.

Now, reduced blood flow to various organs in the body—not only the brain but also the kidneys, intestines, and other organs—has recently been explained in terms of a condition called the *hypercoagulable state.*

According to this theory, an infection, toxin, or stressor—such as an auto accident or surgical procedure—triggers an inflammatory response, which in turn activates a genetically predisposed coagulation process. The so-called "coagulation cascade" leads to the depositing of a protein called *fibrin* onto the lining of vessels all over the body. This process, in turn, results in a decreased supply of oxygen and other blood-borne nutrients to the brain, as well as to other organs such as the kidneys and intestines. The decreased blood and oxygen supplies (termed *ischemia* and *anoxia,* respectively) result in chronic symptoms. In many cases, these symptoms are then associated with a "named" disease such as autism, fibromyalgia, chronic fatigue syndrome, or obsessive-compulsive disorder.

Researchers believe there is a genetic link to the abnormality in coagulation that results in this accumulation of fibrin in the vessel walls. This process doesn't lead to blood clotting in the early stages, because clotting requires a "burst" of thrombin production, and low levels of thrombin elevation just lead to increased fibrin layering. Many autistic individuals also have an elevation of Factor II, a genetic defect associated with the production of fibrin.

For this process to occur, then, you need a genetic predisposition to this condition, along with an inflammatory trigger, such as an infection, trauma, metal or chemical toxin. This triggers an elevation in the level of thrombin, which converts fibrinogen to fibrin. The layering of fibrin in the capillaries results in a decreased flow of oxygen out of the blood and into the brain tissues and other parts of the body. This could help explain why we see decreased blood flow to certain areas of the brain in autistic individuals.

Putting the Immune Puzzle Together

Most people who study immunology do not understand the processes of immunotoxicology, or how toxins affect the immune system. However, this information is essential to our understanding of how autism develops. Children with autism suffer from toxic exposure in early life, which in turn throws their immune systems out of balance. This is in line with research by Anne Connolly at Washington University in St. Louis. Dr. Connolly and her colleagues found autoimmune antibodies to the brain cortex in 36 percent of autistic children, and about 20 percent of Landau-Kleffner children.[24] This is not the root cause of autism, but a secondary process.

Many immunologists point to the immune system characteristics that are aberrant in autistic patients, but very few try to find out why such aberrations occur in the first place. There is no question in my mind that this is an immune-toxicological issue—the damage to the immune system is secondary to heavy metal or xenobiotic toxicity. Now we know that these children have severely elevated levels of toxins in their bodies. How can we possibly ignore this information and continue to focus on secondary factors?

Nutrition, Digestive Dysfunction, and Autism

Every autistic child I have treated suffered from digestive problems and nutritional deficiencies of one kind or another. Here we have not the cause of autism, but another secondary phenomenon in the complex cycle of autistic symptoms.

The question must be asked, Why are so many of these children nutritionally deficient? First, they often have a very limited diet, either because of appetite problems, inadequate attention to giving them a balanced diet, or idiosyncrasies in their food preferences. Second, their systems are working at ten times the rate of a healthy individual. They are trying to detoxify, and they have problems with maldigestion and malabsorption. To make matters worse, their bodies are under tremendous *oxidative stress,* meaning that free radical production and activity have exceeded the body's ability to protect itself against the resulting oxidative damage.

So it is no wonder that autistic children become micronutrient malnourished. With maldigestion, malabsorption, oxidative stress, and a poor diet, how could they not be nutritionally deficient? Does this have anything to do with the root cause of the autism?

The answer is no. These things are not the root cause. They are instead secondary to the toxicity with which these children are suffering. We know this to be true because fixing the digestive problem does not, in turn, fix autism. Pancreatic enzymes, for example, may help these children with their digestive systems, but these enzymes are not going to heal their chronic abnormal brain disease. Again, the cause of this disease begins not in the digestive tract itself but with toxic insults to the digestive organs. It turns out that the liver and pancreas are primary targets of toxic insults from environmental pollutants.[25]

In many cases, autistic children experience food cravings, pica (a craving for nonfood items such as dirt or paint), and other dietary-behavioral problems.[26] Though researchers are not sure what causes these cravings, altered levels of endogenous opioid peptides appear to play a powerful role.[27] These pain-reducing peptides are often elevated in the brains of autistic children.[28] (Note: In a small double-blind clinical trial, drug-induced changes in the opioid system led to favorable changes in immune function in seven of the twelve children who responded; the researchers also recorded a significant reduction in behavioral symptoms associated with autism.[29])

We all know how hard it is to change our eating habits, but for the autistic child this is particularly crucial, since diet can have a direct effect on autistic behavior. Certain foods have been shown to trigger disruptive behavior in autistic children, suggesting a food allergy connection.[30] Some autistic children suffer from reactions or allergies to milk or wheat, creating a whole new set of therapeutic challenges because of the ubiquity of these foods in the typical U.S. diet.

In 2000, a London conference of the Allergy Research Foundation called "Autism: Is It an Allergic Disease?" addressed the complex nutritional processes at work in autism, and their possible connection to food allergies.[31] Their research supports the theory that allergies may be a factor in autism. Antifungal (low-sugar and -yeast), gluten-free, or casein-free diets appear to be effective in treating some of the symptoms seen in autistic children. We should remember, however, that the constellation of factors at work in each autistic patient is unique. What triggers behavioral problems in one child may not be the problem at all for another.

Some autistic children have been found to be deficient in certain vitamins. Low levels of vitamin B_6 (pyridoxine), for example, as well as magnesium and vitamin C (ascorbic acid), have been associated with autism. Supplementation with vitamin C has, in fact, been shown to reduce the severity of autistic symptoms in some children.[32] A number of studies have indicated that combinations of vitamin B_6 and magnesium may offer similar benefits.[33,34,35] Autistic children may also exhibit abnormal blood levels of certain key amino acids, including aspartic acid, glutamate, and taurine.[36] The potential impact of supplementation with these amino acids, however, has yet to be studied in clinical trials. (Please refer back to the amino acid analysis findings of our fourth study, as presented in Chapter 1.)

Autistic children frequently have abnormally low levels of essential trace elements or minerals in their blood—particularly zinc, manganese, and magnesium. These minerals are related to digestion, and deficiencies can impair the secretion of pancreatic enzymes. Of all the trace elements, zinc seems to have the most profound impact on cognitive ability. There is extensive evidence linking zinc and vitamin B_6 deficiencies with a host of behavioral and learning disabilities in children.[37,38,39] Many of zinc's effects center on the hippocampus, a brain tissue site involved in the processing of memory, cognition, and integration of emotion.[40] According to one theory, a fetus developing in the womb of a zinc-deficient pregnant woman may experience a major disruption in the normal development of the brain; this may later develop into autism in the infant or young child.[41]

Clinically low levels of magnesium in blood plasma are associated with states of hyperexcitability and inattention in children. Venezuelan scientists reported in the December 1988 *Archives of Environmental Health* that the hair of forty mentally retarded children showed significantly low levels of magnesium, as well as iron and copper.[42] Magnesium, along with copper, plays an active role in mobilizing the ATP-enzyme system on which virtually all of the body (and brain) cells' energy depends. Nutritionist Mildred Seelig, former director of the American College of Nutrition, has estimated that 80 to 90 percent of the U.S. population may have a magnesium deficiency. Marginal deficiencies of zinc, copper, and manganese may be widespread as well.[43]

At least eleven trace elements—copper, iron, zinc, cobalt, iodine, molybdenum, manganese, magnesium, selenium, chromium, and fluorine—have been recognized as essential for human development and overall health.

Most of these are built into key enzymes and hormones; some function as ions (charged atoms) affecting tissue contractility and blood pH balance. Still others are used in the brain's production of neurotransmitters, chemical messengers necessary for proper brain function. Many elements are stored in the bone and in organs which serve as reservoirs in times of chronic deficiency. There is now substantial evidence that the effects of trace elements on the brain can result in significant improvements in mental processes.[44,45,46]

Digestive weaknesses (e.g., malabsorption) can promote many of the mineral deficiencies we see in children with neurodevelopmental problems. In treating autistic children, however, it's important to remember that elemental deficits in the body do not always stem from clear-cut dietary deficiencies. Diets high in the simple sugars sucrose and fructose reduce the body's ability to utilize and retain copper and chromium—the very elements it needs to control blood sugar. Many anemia cases may have less to do with dietary iron than with deficiencies of vitamin C, which greatly boosts iron absorption. Similarly, a low zinc level may sometimes be caused by a high-protein diet. Copper, cadmium, and lead, when present in excess, tend to deplete the body's zinc supply—which makes sense in light of our findings that many of our autistic patients are deficient in zinc and have high levels of cadmium, lead, and other heavy metals.

As I have mentioned, the urine of autistic children has also been shown to be high in peptides. Many autistic children suffer from "leaky gut" syndrome. In one study of twenty-one autistic children compared with forty normal controls, nine of the twenty-one were found to have abnormal intestinal permeability, while none of the controls did. The researchers speculate that peptides may pass through the intestinal walls of these children, leading to behavioral abnormalities.[47] They can cross through the gut into the bloodstream, cross the blood-brain barrier, and damage the brain.

The Liver Link with Autism

My research has confirmed that there is a congenital defect in liver detoxication in all of the autistic spectrum disorders. In an earlier study by Waring, 90 percent of the autistics examined were deficient in phenosulfotransferase, a liver enzyme that plays a key role in detoxication.[48] Consequently, toxic substances that can lead to abnormalities in the brain accumulate in the bodies of these children.

For a healthy individual, exposure to ordinary environmental chemicals like paints, plastics, glues, and carpets doesn't normally present any difficulty, unless there is a massive exposure. For the individual with a dysfunctional liver detoxication system, however, these ordinary chemical exposures can be devastating.

The functions of the liver and brain are interdependent. Impaired liver detoxication has been linked to both cognitive and emotional impairments.[49] The two phases of liver detoxication must be balanced for an individual to be mentally and emotionally healthy.

In essence, with pathological detoxication, the liver becomes a major *contributor* to the toxic burden, rather than the organ that normally alleviates this burden. It's like a water filter that has suddenly become so clogged with pollutants that the "drinking water" that comes out is dirtier than what went in. The result of pathological detoxication is a rapid buildup of free radicals and toxic substances in the bodies of autistic children. This explains, in a nutshell, why these children accumulate neurotoxins and immunotoxins far more easily than other children.

Let's take a closer look at different aspects of pathological detoxication. When the liver's two key detox phases are out of balance, certain nutritional deficiencies can exacerbate the problem. A high-fat junk food diet lacking in natural fibers (which help clear out the digestive tract) and fresh vegetables increases the burden on the liver. In particular, certain nutrients help stimulate phase II activity, including phenolic acids, coumarins, dithiolethiones, and thiocarbamates—all of which are primarily found in vegetables.[50] The richest sources for these nutrients are cruciferous vegetables, such as broccoli, kale, collards, cabbage, and brussels sprouts.[51] Turmeric and N-acetyl cysteine (a precursor to the potent antioxidant glutathione) can also help stimulate the liver's phase II system.

When the liver isn't detoxifying normally, lipophilic (literally, "fat-loving") xenobiotic chemicals are not properly metabolized. So these lipophilic compounds pass directly into the brain, at a developmental juncture when the blood-brain barrier cannot protect developing brain structures. The result is damage to neurons, dendritic processes, receptors, and mitochondrial DNA. Toxic xenobiotic chemicals can damage and activate enzymes in the cell called 2'S A-synthetase and PKR (protein kinase), which in turn leads to a decrease in the production of messenger RNA (mRNA).

Now, when mRNA is deficient, cells do not manufacture proteins. This is Biology 101. In the case of the central nervous system, this leads to the failure to produce key structures in the nervous system, such as tubulin, axial fibrillary proteins, and dendrites. Neuronal protein production may also be thrown off. These factors alone can lead to the dysfunction of cerebral and cerebellar functions, yielding the complex variety of behaviors seen in the autistic spectrum of disorders. In addition to the direct injury, an activated immune system brought on by toxic xenobiotic injury reacts to injured autogenic components, creating a syndrome of autoimmune neurotoxicity.

To compound the problem, autistic children have been found to have abnormally low levels of sulphates in their blood, an indication that their detoxifying capacities are deficient.[52] Sulphate molecules act as conjugators for phase II, enabling the excretion of these toxins from the body. In one study, 232 children with autism compared with 86 controls were found to have low blood levels of sulphates, and high sulphate levels in urine, compared with controls.[53] When the level of sulphates in the blood is too low, the body may retain toxins, which can then damage the nervous system. Low levels of sulphates are also associated with gut dysfunction, increased gut permeability, and inflammation. Autistic children who have low sulphate levels may consequently have lower levels of secretin, and therefore essential pancreatic enzymes may be blocked.[54]

A genetic defect in the liver detoxication process, then, appears to contribute to neurotoxicity by generating the development of molecular injuries to parts of the central nervous system, which in turn may damage the development of other pathways and systems in the body. Which specific pathways are most affected by this process at certain developmental junctures may explain the clusters of different functional anomalies we find in the autistic spectrum disorders.

A congenital defect in the liver detoxication system, along with food allergies, a nutritionally poor diet, maldigestion, and malabsorption—all contribute to this picture of toxicity. The greater the lack of essential nutrients, the more difficult it is for the liver to detoxify xenobiotic chemicals. All these factors create a vicious circle that tips the body further and further out of balance, bringing a heavy "total load" burden of toxicity to bear on the body's weakened systems. This cycle is what leads to the behavioral manifestation of autistic symptoms.

Understanding the Neurotoxic Syndrome

Toxic damage to the nervous system, or neurotoxicity, is caused by three factors—environmental exposure (gestation or postgestational) to toxic substances, abnormal liver detoxication, and nutritional deficiencies. Environmental exposure to toxic environmental chemicals and heavy metals leads to the production of free radicals, which can then damage the brain. As we have seen, toxic exposure also throws the immune system off balance, and this leads to the production of autoimmune antibodies to the brain. All this damage causes brain fragments to circulate in the body, which further stimulates the immune system.

All of this leads to other kinds of neurotoxic injuries. Neurons and mitochondria are damaged. When 2'5A synthetase is activated, mRNA production decreases, leading to further injury of receptors and dendrites, as well as abnormal kinase production. This in turn causes dysfunction in intercerebral and intercerebellar areas, which we find in the autistic spectrum disorders.

These are some of the ways that exposure to toxic agents can indirectly inflict damage to the central nervous system. Exposure to these agents can also permanently damage neurons and brain processes, changes which are evident from PET scans and autopsies of autistic individuals.

The Effects of Chemical Pollutants

Now let's look at how some of these toxic agents directly affect the nervous system. When we test autistic children for the presence of heavy metals and xenobiotic chemicals, we frequently find elevated levels of chemicals such as hexane and pentane, as well as elevated levels of heavy metals such as mercury and lead. We know that autistic children harbor high—often dangerously high—levels of these substances in their bodies, but how exactly do their neurotoxic effects contribute to the etiology of this disorder?

Take hexane, a chemical derived from crude oil and used as a solvent to help dissolve other chemicals in industrial processes. Hexane enters the air, water, and food chain during its manufacture and use. It can enter the environment through spills, evaporation, or landfills. Gasoline, automobile exhaust, and cooking oils are also common sources of exposure. People who work in certain industries, such as shoe manufacturing, printing, or construction, are especially at risk of exposure.

Hexane can enter the body through air, water, skin exposure, or food. Once it is in the body, it goes to all the organs of the body. If it gets to the liver and the liver is functioning efficiently, then the liver through various mechanisms tends to dispose of it into the intestinal tract or into the urine through the kidneys. The problem arises when the liver is functioning inefficiently. At that point, not all of the hexane gets out of the body, but is returned to areas of the body that have high fat content. In addition, there are intermediate metabolites formed which are free radicals, and which are released from the liver to damage almost any organ system.

The neurotoxic effects of hexane are, of course, more severe for a developing fetus than for a full-grown adult. Again, fetal brain cells are much more vulnerable than fully developed and protected adult brain cells. So the timing of the exposure has a lot to do with its effects on the body. If the fetus is exposed to a high dose of hexane, it can disrupt all kinds of neurodevelopmental processes.

(For physicians and researchers, these changes in the central nervous system after hexane exposure, mostly visible only with an electron microscope, are as follows: First, one sees accumulations of neurofilaments in the swollen axons. These filaments are not lining up properly and may be forming tangled masses. There is also a disruption of the mitochondria and neurotubules, as well as pronounced swelling of the endoneurial tissue. In addition, there is fiber degeneration in the nerve trunks. In the central nervous system there is damage to the white matter of the cerebellum, cerebrum, and brain stem. Imagine the damage that could occur in the vulnerable nervous system of a three-week-old fetus exposed to a massive amount of hexane.)

We also find elevated levels of hexane in the bodies of all types of patients with chronic illnesses, including autism and other developmental disorders, lupus and other autoimmune diseases, ALS, Parkinson's disease, chronic fatigue syndrome, ADHD, multiple sclerosis, and possibly Alzheimer's disease. Hexane is probably only one of the factors in the development of these diseases.

There have been many theories concerning the cause of hexane's damaging effects on the nervous system. Spencer suggests hexane exposure leads to enzyme inhibitions vital to glycolysis. This would result in a reduction of energy production needed for normal neuronal function. All of this may lead to neuronal malfunctioning, axonal degeneration, and even loss of neurons. Other theories: Graham suggests that hexane exposure relates to cross-linking of neurofilaments. Savolainen says the cause relates to the solvents being transferred to reactive metabolites, leading to denaturation of proteins. And according to a fourth theory, hexane exposure may cause alterations in the formation of cholesterol in the cell membranes of nerve tissue, therefore impairing neuronal function.

This gives you a snapshot of the neurotoxic process caused by one xenobiotic chemical, a toxin that likely contributes to the development of this illness in some autistic children. I should note that two other common environmental chemicals, 2-methyl pentane and 3-methyl pentane (both isomers of hexane), have effects in the human body that are virtually identical to those of hexane. Other chemicals, such as organophosphates, chlorinated hydrocarbons, and others, may have a similar net result, with myriad damaging effects on the nervous system.

The Effects of Heavy Metal Pollutants

In my autistic patients I also often find elevated levels of certain heavy metals—most often mercury, lead, and tin—which, like hexane and pentane, are known to be potent neurotoxins. In our study of fifty-four autistic children, sixteen out of fifty-four had significant elevations (above 10 mcg per liter) of mercury; twenty-one out of fifty-four had elevated lead; and eighteen of fifty-four had elevated tin.

Free radicals are generated as by-products of both heavy metal and toxic chemical exposures. These free radicals may account for much of the nerve-damaging effects of toxic metals, since nerve cell membranes are so vulnerable to the damaging effects of free radicals.

Heavy metal poisoning may produce widespread systemic signs in addition to central nervous disturbances, making the diagnosis of a toxic metal disorder readily apparent. Though we know a lot about how mercury affects the nervous system, the mechanisms of other heavy metals are not so easily found (though we do have some research on tin and lead).

It is no accident that in many cases we find abnormally high levels of mercury, sometimes at alarmingly elevated levels, in our autistic patients. Autism has been identified in some cases as an unrecognized mercurial syndrome, a case of undiagnosed mercury poisoning. Indeed, mercury toxicity symptoms are similar to those of autism, on the behavioral, bio-chemical, and molecular levels.[55] Nonetheless only one out of every three autistic children I've studied displays mercury toxicity.

Erethism, or the syndrome of organic metal disturbances seen in chronic inorganic mercury poisoning, is characterized by irritability, difficulty concentrating, and insomnia. Affected persons often suffer from overwhelming tiredness, extreme timidity, shyness, embarrassment, discouragement, and apathy. Memory loss and cognitive impairments usually accompany the disorder. Hallucinations and seizures may also occur. Although psychiatric symptoms may be the earliest manifestation of intoxication, gingivitis, dermatitis, and tremor are also characteristic features of inorganic mercury exposure.

In the case of autism, we are talking here about the low-level, chronic, long-term accumulation of mercury, not large acute exposure (that's a different subject). Most of the problem with mercury toxicity is its indolent, slow, smoldering effects that damage neurons slowly but incrementally. Rarely would a physician who lacks training in environmental medicine suspect that mercury is at the root of the problem. Exposure to mercury begins in the womb where the mother transfers mercury to the fetus through the placenta. Once the fetus is out of the uterus, there are many ways for mercury levels to begin to accumulate.

Why do some people become mercury toxic? This is a question of how much "goes in" versus what "goes out." If more goes in than goes out, there is a buildup, so the exposure is important. There are natural ways the body gets rid of mercury. One of these involves conjugation of the potent antioxidant compound (classified by biochemists as a tripeptide aminothiol) in our body called *glutathione*. Also, the amino acid cysteine will also form a complex with mercury to remove it. In general, we have a balance between how much gets into the body and how much we eliminate and the end result is what is stored in the brain, liver, and kidneys. Genetic defects in the metabolic pathways involved in this process may also play a role. The bottom line is that mercury toxicity is far more complicated than just being exposed to mercury.

Mercury damages the blood-brain barrier. It is neurotoxic and thus damages nerve cells. Mercury also generates free radicals that go on to damage nerve cells. There is an excess of oxidative stress and the depletion of glutathione and other thiols, causing increased neurotoxicity from interactions of reactive oxygen species, glutamate, and dopamine. It is well known for destroying the tubulin protein structure in the neuron, and also inhibits the production of neurotransmitters. It does this by inhibiting calcium-dependent neurotransmitter release.

How does mercury enter the body of a child? A pregnant woman with elevated levels of elemental mercury transfers it directly to her fetus in very large quantities both through the placenta and through breast milk. If the detoxication system for the removal of mercury is efficient, some of the mercury leaves via the stool and some through the urine. A very small amount also leaves through the lungs.

An important point that must be remembered is that the fetus, up until about 18 months of life, does not have a protective blood-brain barrier and so a much larger amount of mercury can get into the brain during these most vulnerable periods than at other times.

As I introduced in Chapter 3, lead is the other heavy metal that has exacted a heavy toll on our children's mental health. Like mercury, lead has long been known to have neurotoxic effects, and can cross the blood-brain barrier. Like mercury, lead can be stored in the mother's body for years before it is activated and passed on to the fetus during gestation or breastfeeding. Lead is particularly known for causing cognitive impairments.

Although severe intoxication with inorganic lead has long been recognized as a cause of brain damage in adults, the more subtle effects of lower level intoxications in adults have been elucidated only in the past decade. Severe depression, anxiety, sleep disorders, irritability, fatigue, difficulties in concentration, and memory loss can all be a result of intoxication with inorganic lead. Because not all lead-intoxicated patients with depression or other psychiatric features will suffer from other classic features of intoxication, such as anemia, colic, or peripheral neuropathies, a history of exposure to inorganic lead is the most important clue to the diagnosis. Depressive symptoms may be severe enough to meet the criteria for a major depression, but the disorder is best characterized as an organic affective disorder, which places proper emphasis on the etiologic significance or intoxication with inorganic lead. Exposure to other metals may also lead to severe neuropsychiatric symptoms.

Lead poisoning has been identified as a contributing factor in the pathology of infantile autism.[56] In addition, many studies have shown correlations between lead poisoning and lowered IQ, learning disabilities, developmental disorders, and impaired motor skills. A group of rural children who were mildly retarded or of borderline intelligence tested higher for lead and cadmium than normal controls, even though all the children's exposure levels were considered to be subtoxic.[57]

As with other toxins, the extent and nature of the neurotoxic damage caused by lead depends on the timing and dose of exposure, as well as the genetic predisposition of the individual child. Low-level exposure to lead, either *in utero* or during the first few years of life, is significantly associated with cognitive impairment, mental disorders, hyperactivity, attention deficit disorders, and other behavioral problems.[58,59]

From this discussion we can conclude that exposure to these and other heavy metals—which are highly toxic even for adults—can seriously damage and disrupt the developing nervous system in a fetus or infant, leading to all sorts of problems later in life. We do not yet understand the mechanisms by which this neurotoxic damage results in autistic spectrum disorders. But the consistently high levels of these substances that we find in autistic children should be telling us something—that their neurotoxic effects likely play a role in the etiology of this illness.

Autism as a Systemic Disease

Modern medicine, with its predominant focus on eliminating symptoms and interfering with the superficial mechanisms of disease, is ill equipped to handle autism and other chronic neurodevelopmental disorders. According to the traditional allopathic treatment paradigm, infection is the primary cause of illness. This worked fine earlier in the twentieth century when that was the case. But the epidemic rise of chronic illnesses we are now seeing is related to increasing low-level exposure to chemical and heavy metal toxicity in the environment.

Most of the chronic diseases that traditional medicine has no idea how to treat are related to these low-level toxic exposures that people are accumulating, because of poor nutrition and the fact that their livers are being depleted of these nutrients and aren't functioning efficiently. People are building up these toxins in their bodies, so that by the time they're forty or fifty or sixty years old, they come down with some chronic degenerative disease, whether it is mediated by the immune system or the central nervous system. This is the new paradigm of disease as I see it.

Autism is multifaceted—many organ systems are involved. A complex web of interrelationships connects areas of injury and things that are inflicting injury. In my studies (discussed in Chapter 1) I have shown that toxic chemicals are present in these children; and that the kids have abnormal liver detoxication characteristics. Autism is both an environmental and a genetic defect. The autistic children I have treated have an abnormal liver detoxication that is a genetic process.

The basic problem of autism is actually quite simple. We live in an environment that is toxic, and these particular children simply cannot get rid of toxins that other children manage to neutralize and eliminate. The autistic children I've studied consistently show elevated levels of xenobiotic chemicals and metals in their tissues damaging various organ systems, especially the developing brain, which primarily attracts lipophilic xenobiotic chemicals. In addition, the immune system gets damaged, leading to many secondary effects. It has become abundantly clear that autism is a *systemic disease* affecting almost any organ system including the pancreas, kidneys, liver, intestinal tract, and of course, the brain.

Monica's Story

I first met Monica, the little girl I introduced in Chapter 2 of this book, in March 1996, when she was five years old. Monica's somber manner belied her soft babyish looks, her wispy hair, and deep-set blue eyes. The day her mother brought her to my office, she carefully avoided eye contact with me, and did not speak, making only a tuneless humming noise. She kept her eyes fixed on a colorful mobile that hung from the ceiling near the window in my office. There was something fragile about her, as though her very survival depended on her silence and remoteness.

Two years earlier, at the age of three, Monica had stopped speaking entirely. Around that time she had been diagnosed with severe autism. She would scream with terror when her parents tried to touch her or interact with her. She reacted with terror whenever there was a change in routine—when her parents bought her a new dress, or when they took a different route than usual home from the grocery store. She spent most of her time playing silently with her stuffed animals in her room, rearranging them in tidy rows, and this was the only activity that seemed to calm her.

Since her diagnosis, Monica's parents had taken her to see at least ten doctors—from pediatric neurologists to child psychologists. They had tried behavioral therapy, sensory integration therapy, special diets, all manner of nutritional supplements, and homeopathy. But in spite of all of it, Monica only seemed to retreat further and further into her own world.

The first thing I did was to take a thorough history and do a physical examination. Monica's parents filled out an elaborate questionnaire that detailed not only her health history, but anything in their own histories that might have contributed to toxic exposure. We were looking for clues, however obscure, that might shed light on the cause of this disease.

The next stage was to test Monica for heavy metals and other toxins, as well as digestion and liver function. Right away we found that her mercury levels were severely elevated. The tests also revealed abnormally high levels of lead and tin. In addition, we found that her liver function was compromised. Tests showed elevated D-glucaric and mercapturic acid levels, indicating chemical toxicity. She also suffered from malabsorption, maldigestion, and nutritional deficiencies.

As it turned out, Monica—like all of the autistic children I have treated—also suffered from multiple allergies. Her skin and blood tests revealed food, inhalant, and chemical sensitivities. The blood studies revealed IgE and IgG-type allergic responses, as well as T-cell changes.

Monica's family lived in Vermont, so we were able to begin her treatment right away with the help of a local M.D. We began with detoxification therapy, which included the removal of heavy metals from her body. In Monica's case, her severely elevated level of mercury was what concerned us most. This was treated with DMPS chelation therapy twice a week by a physician in another state.

Monica began to improve within two months of the DMPS therapy. A subtle change became apparent. Slowly, she grew more alert. She would look her parents in the eye, and seemed to listen when they spoke to her. Soon she began to speak again. Everyone in her world was amazed at the occurrence. Also, we improved the receptiveness, and the abnormal behaviors disappeared. Over the eighteen months following her first nine months of DMPS therapy, she continued to improve from 50 to 85 percent.

I last saw Monica in 2001. I would say that she is almost 100% improved since the first time I met her. Her only impairment is the ability to abstract. Overall, you cannot determine if she is autistic from looking at her, talking to her, or watching her. You would have to perform specific neurometric or psychological tests to recognize the continued present abnormalities—they are so subtle, it is amazing. We tested Monica again for toxins and found that she continues to have chemical toxicity and heavy metal toxicity. My clinical experience indicates this is because her parents have been unable to maintain consistent and aggressive treatment.

Monica's teacher Alice and I arranged to meet with her after school to perform a short interview to test her progress. We met at a field near her school. Monica was already at the field with her mother when we arrived, smiling and laughing, swinging on the swing set with two of her friends. Her mother called her over to say hello.

"Hi Monica! Are those your friends from school?" Alice asks.

"Yes." Monica looks straight into Alice's eyes.

"What are their names?"

"Vikram and . . . Julia."

"Are you going to a skating party?" Alice asks her.

"Yes. At Julia's house."

Monica and Alice talked more about school. Monica said she doesn't like to do math in school, but she likes to draw pictures in her journal.

Alice's next question was one of Monica's favorites. "What do you want to be when you grow up?"

"A doctor," Monica said instantly. "With a Ferrari and a big house," she continued. "A *mansion*." This is a girl who, in 1996, would not utter a word or look anyone in the eye.

"Now may I interview *you*?" Monica asked with a smile, and Alice nodded. But just then Monica's friends called to her. She jumped up and waved to us gaily as she ran off to join them.

Chapter 6

◆

The Distortion of Development

In the preceding chapter I attempted to show how autism is far more than just a neurological or behavioral disorder. I gave you a glimpse of the complexity of this disorder, how the dysfunction of certain organ systems in the body creates a vicious cycle of toxic burden. I showed how the developing brain and central nervous system are the unfortunate victims of this toxic buildup.

My colleagues and I have documented the immune, digestive, and detoxication problems in these children. At this point, we might well ask, What triggers this cascade of harmful reactions in the first place? Where does it all begin?

Autistic behavior may not be detected until an infant is at least around eighteen months old. Nonetheless, the chain of events leading to the autistic syndrome begins much earlier. My own research has convinced me that this disease has its roots in three key phases prior to birth: (1) the preconception period, when either the father's sperm or the mother's egg is damaged; (2) during embryonic development, the first few weeks of gestation; or (3) throughout pregnancy, with ongoing exposure to neurotoxic substances during fetal life.

Please keep in mind that this is only a theory, albeit one based on established science. More study is needed to verify the mechanisms I propose. I am quite confident, however, that my theory helps explain the roots of autism more comprehensively than ever before.

First, let's take a look at how environmental toxins may harm the parents' germ cells—the egg and sperm—prior to conception.

Damaged Seed, Damaged Child

A parent's exposure to toxic substances prior to conception can throw off the normal course of neurological development. As the world becomes more toxic, I believe that preconceptional planning, with an eye toward maximizing the health of both the father and the mother, will become increasingly important in order to lower the risk of autism and other neuro-developmental problems.

In the large-scale 1975 study coordinated by the National Institutes of Health, researchers examined the relationship between certain environmental factors and autism. Women who had the most occupational exposure to chemicals *prior to conception* gave birth more often to autistic children than mothers who were not exposed to such chemicals. Based on this finding, it seems logical to conclude that injury to the egg or sperm can lead to autism as well as a host of other neurodevelopmental disorders.

A healthy male produces millions of new sperm cells every day. This rapid production may make the sperm especially vulnerable to toxic damage. Indeed, many chemicals are known to substantially alter sperm counts and cause sperm abnormalities. In one study, when seven-day-old male mice were injected with parathion, a chemical used in pesticides, their sperm counts decreased and DNA was altered. The animals' sperm was damaged twenty-eight to fifty days after exposure to the pesticides.[1] Parathion is one of many pesticides that can cause cytotoxic and genetic alterations in germ cells.

Other substances showing toxic effects on sperm that could potentially lead to fetal abnormalities include heavy metals and various forms of air pollution, notably cigarette smoke.[2,3] Heavy metals such as lead, cadmium, and aluminum also have toxic effects on sperm,[4] as does methyl-mercury.[5] Copper is commonly imbalanced in people with inflammatory conditions and excessive oxidative stress, and high copper levels are also associated with damaged sperm. In one study of impala living close to a copper mine, high copper levels were correlated with significant sperm abnormalities (in particular, sperm with neck vacuoles).[6]

Exposure to lead is particularly harmful to sperm, and likely reduces one's fertility as well. Lead apparently does more than simply suppress sperm counts. Researchers have found that lead alters sperm function by affecting the hormonal control of sperm production, rather than by direct toxic action on sperm.[7] In one study, battery workers exposed to high levels of airborn lead were shown to have abnormal sperm counts.[8] Diesel exhaust and many other chemicals have been shown to reduce sperm motility.[9]

Many other drugs and chemicals have been shown to have toxic effects on sperm and on the generation of new sperm, spermatogenesis.[10] Xylene, one of the chemicals we measure in autistic children, induces morphological abnormalities in sperm.[11] High xylene levels would tend to be more common in people living around areas of urban pollution or heavy industry.

Free radicals, those highly reactive and unstable molecules I introduced earlier, also immobilize and damage sperm.[12] Although free radicals can come from a wide variety of sources, the two most prolific sources in modern lifestyles are high-fat diets and exposure to tobacco smoke. Linoleic acid, perhaps the most commonly consumed of all dietary fats (actually referred to as a fatty acid), has been shown to reduce sperm motility.[13] Ironically, much of the problem with high-fat foods may have less to do with the fat itself than with all the chemicals that are concentrated in that fat—pesticides, xylene, and many others.

Smoking is a gargantuan source of free radicals, with each puff carrying hundreds of billions of these destructive molecules. This may explain, in part, why smoking can lead to chromosome errors in both ova and sperm, which can impact reproductive outcomes.[14] Cigarette tobacco also contains cadmium, nicotine, cotinine (a metabolite of nicotine), and other toxic chemicals—all potentially damaging to the sperm. Cigarette smoke also dramatically decreases sperm motility, a fairly good sign that the sperm are suffering the consequences of toxic overload.[15]

Could it be that our standard American diet, combined with exposure to smoke and other forms of air pollution, is exacting a heavy toll on our reproductive health? I have little doubt that this is indeed the case. Some researchers have suggested that the fall in sperm counts all over the world is linked to the presence of xenobiotic chemicals in the environment, and particularly the estrogen-like effects of some of these chemicals.[16]

Other xenobiotic chemicals are found to be particularly harmful to the ovum. One pervasive chemical we have found elevated levels of in our autistic patients, hexachlorobenzene, is known to be destructive to ovarian germ cells.[17] It seems entirely possible that if the infant or young child has accumulated this chemical, the parents had prior exposure as well.

Researchers aren't sure yet exactly how exposures of the egg or sperm to certain chemicals and heavy metals influence fetal development, or how they may be related to autism. What we do know is that many xenobiotic chemicals and heavy metals inflict damage to both sperm and ova. Because of a growing body of compelling research in this area, more rigorous standards have been developed in recent years for determining prenatal toxicity.[18]

A Toxic Womb

Once the egg has been fertilized, the arduous journey to the creation of a healthy, normally functioning human being begins. During pregnancy (gestation), the prenatal brain is constantly becoming more complex, adding new cells, connections, and special areas—all forming increasingly intricate networks of communication. Anything that disrupts this normal process of brain development can have a devastating effect on the sensory, social, language, and mental functions of an individual.

During fetal life, because the blood-brain barrier is not yet in place, many of the harmful chemicals to which a mother is exposed—even substances to which she may have been exposed years prior to conception—can be mobilized and passed on to the fetus. The manifestation of autistic behavior varies from one individual to another, depending on the amount and toxicity of the chemicals and heavy metals to which the fragile central nervous system is exposed, and at what stage of development the exposure occurs.

I believe the critical event that triggers autism is an exposure to significant levels of neurotoxins during this extremely vulnerable period in neurological development. Since the blood-brain barrier does not form until an infant is about six months old, the fetal brain, then, has no protective tissue to keep these toxins out. During gestation, the prenatal brain is developing rapidly, and exposure to neurotoxins in this early period can disrupt brain function in fundamental and even in permanent ways.

Our knowledge of exactly how and when this damage occurs, however, and how it leads to autism, is still very limited. Neuroscientists need to elucidate the precise mechanisms at work in this process. Let's take a look at what we do know about toxic injury during early life, and how it relates to the autistic spectrum.

The fetus can be exposed to environmental toxins through the mother in several ways. Toxins may be passed from mother to fetus or infant four different ways—through the placenta, skin, respiratory tract, and gastrointestinal tract.[19] The infant may also be exposed to toxins through the mother's breast milk. These toxins may even reach levels higher in the fetus or infant's blood than in the mother's.

Timing and the ability of the liver to detoxify are the most crucial factors in determining the outcome in such a situation. It is clear that we are dealing with both an environmental and a genetic problem. If a mother during her pregnancy comes in contact with the toxic chemical hexane, for example, hexane goes directly into the fetus. If the fetus has an efficient detoxication system, the hexane will leave the fetus as fast as it came in, as long as there isn't a massive exposure.

But let us consider another scenario. Let's say the mother and fetus experience a moderate exposure to hexane. At the same time, the fetus has a genetic defect in certain critical aspects of liver detoxication. Early in fetal life, when the central nervous system is in the developmental stages and there is no blood-brain barrier present as there is in an adult, we find that the brain can easily succumb to toxic insults. This can lead to all sorts of developmental aberrations of the brain. The exact type of damage incurred in the central nervous system depends on genetics, and also on the haphazard nature of the damage inflicted by both the toxins and the harmful free radicals they form.

This toxicity then leads to damaged signaling and lack of receptor transmission. Toxins can also damage thousands of key enzyme systems which, together with the failure of molecular signaling mechanisms, leads to aberrant brain function—the autistic brain.

In an adult, of course, we do not see the same type of damage that we see in the developing brain. Again, this is simply because fetal brain cells are much more vulnerable than fully developed and protected adult brain cells.

I am not the only one to propose that this disorder has its roots, at least in part, during fetal life. This theory has gained credence among some researchers with an understanding of neurotoxic phenomena. According to Christopher Gillberg and Mary Coleman, authors of *The Biology of the Autistic Syndromes,* autism appears to be the result of a specific disease process that usually occurs, or begins, in utero. And the nature of the impairments we find in autistic children can give us clues about when during gestation this injury likely occurred.

During the first and second trimesters of development, the fetus is particularly vulnerable to injury that may lead to autism.[20] Abnormal development of the nervous system results in "neural misconnection," which in turn gives rise to autistic behavior.[21]

Autistic children with abnormal facial features are thought to have suffered some kind of injury during the first trimester of pregnancy, a period when the facial features are still developing.[22] Autism resulting from thalidomide exposure during the first trimester, between the twentieth and twenty-fourth days of gestation, is one example of this phenomenon.

We also know that problems with cortical development tend to occur during the second trimester.[23] Autistic children with normal faces and bodies likely have undergone some trauma during the second trimester, once the face is already fully formed. "High functioning" autistic individuals or those with Asperger's syndrome tend to exhibit neurological abnormalities that point to some injury or insult during the second trimester.

Another important clue to how all of this fits together is that many of the structural brain abnormalities associated with autism appear in areas of the brain that develop during the fifth week of gestation. These include a whole slew of changes that are often described by highly technical and even esoteric-sounding terms. Here are the main changes: reduced numbers of Purkinje neurons; agenesis of the superior olive; dysgenesis of the facial nucleus; increased neuron-packing density of the medial, cortical, and central nuclei of the amygdala and medium septum; and hypoplasia of the brainstem and posterior cerebellum.[24] (An explanation of each of these changes is clearly beyond the scope of this book. I list them here for those of you who would like to share the information with a neurobiologist or developmental psychiatrist.)

Whenever the disruption of development may occur, it is evident that some form of injury in early life triggers autism. Because the exact nature of this insult—whether caused by exposure to toxic agents, or infection, or some other factor—is different in every case, diagnosis and treatment are also highly individual. As Gillberg and Coleman put it, autism is not one syndrome but many syndromes, each one being the individual outcome of a complex process triggered by some kind of injury to the developing nervous system.

The Neurotoxic Barrage: Heavy Metals Revisited

What kinds of toxic substances pose the greatest risk to the fragile developing nervous system? I've described a number of these in preceding chapters. Researchers are now beginning to identify the main culprits behind the neurotoxic phenomenon of autism. As I've noted, we humans are most vulnerable to the neurotoxic effects of xenobiotic chemicals and heavy metals during gestation and early infancy. Even toxins to which the mother has been exposed long *before conception* can be passed on to the infant, as these are often stored up in the mother's body fat. PCBs, lead, and mercury can all be passed on in this way.[25] Additionally, in the United States, one out of ten newborns (about 375,000 a year) is exposed to illegal recreational drugs in the womb.

We have already seen that heavy metals such as lead, mercury, cadmium, and tin have dramatic neurotoxic effects. Prenatal exposure to seven heavy metals—cadmium, tin, cobalt, lead, mercury, nickel, and silver—has been shown to have toxic effects on the fetus; the higher the exposure, the greater the cognitive skill impairments and the greater the frequency of childhood illnesses.[26]

Exposure to toxic metals has also been associated with depression, learning and behavioral impairments, mental retardation, autism and other developmental disorders, violence, and lowered IQ. Heavy metal toxicity is thought to explain as much as 20 percent of the cognitive differences among children in the same age group with low levels of exposure to toxic metals.

Methylmercury is the form of mercury most likely to be associated with the risk for developmental effects. As with many toxins, exposure to methylmercury can come through gestation or breastfeeding. The effects on the infant may be very subtle or more pronounced. It all depends on the degree of exposure, as well as the genetic expression of that exposure (the body's built-in response to it). In cases where the exposure may be minimal, there may not even be anything detected like a small decrease in IQ. It might be necessary to use sophisticated neuropsychological testing tools to determine the minor effects that mercury has had on the brain.

In cases of more severe exposure, the effects may be very serious but they may be delayed. The infant, as in many cases of the autistic spectrum, may be born normally only to show the significant changes at a later time. The delays may not come until parents notice delays in the milestones of development like walking and talking. We see this in the autistic spectrum of disorders all the time. The very serious effects such as blindness, deafness, inability to walk or speak, and seizures are usually associated with very severe toxic exposures. Classic examples of such catastrophes include two famous accidents involving mercury: the Minimata disaster in

Japan, where mercury was being dumped into the water near a fishing village, and the contamination of massive amounts of grain in Iraq, grain that was used to make bread.

I have devoted a great deal of time and energy to studying the potential role of mercury in neurotoxic damage. Mercury exposure leads to abnormal hormone levels, disrupting development and irreversibly damaging the nervous system. One study of ninety-two pregnant women examined the effect of exposure to various heavy metals at about seventeen weeks gestation. In follow-up tests on their children (at age three), the higher the toxic exposure during fetal life, the worse were these children's performance on the McCarthy Scales of Children's Abilities, and the higher their rates of childhood illness.[27]

Lead also has a particularly toxic effect on the developing nervous system, since it interferes with certain biochemical activity that depends on calcium ions, as well as neuronal connections dependent on dendritic pruning.[28] Exposure to lead and other toxic substances has also been associated directly with autism. Fetal exposure to lead is correlated with low socioeconomic status, exposure to old houses with lead paint, and poor nutrition (especially deficiencies in calcium, iron, and zinc).

Gillberg and Coleman have noted that in cases of lead poisoning, it is often difficult to tell whether the lead poisoning caused the autism, or whether the autism occurred first. Though in some cases lead poisoning may be irreversible, chelation therapy may help alleviate autistic symptoms in some children who are born with lead poisoning. Children with autism also appear to be at greater risk for repeated exposure to lead poisoning, which of course contributes to the vicious cycle of toxic overload.

On a biochemical level, heavy metals are known to deplete certain key antioxidants, such as glutathione, resulting in production of harmful free radicals that also damage the brain and nervous system, and contribute to autoimmune conditions. Heavy metals also affect synaptic transmission in the brain and nervous system. They disrupt calcium levels in the brain and in cells, which affect many functions—CNS function, cognition, and release of certain key neurotransmitters (serotonin, norepinephrine, acetylcholine) that affect mood and motivation.

Heavy metals also tend to underlie many forms of nutritional imbalance. These metals disrupt the balances of key micronutrients (vitamins and minerals), such as zinc, iron, magnesium, lithium, vitamin B_6, and vitamin B_{12}. When these nutrients are depleted, they can't effectively serve the brain; nor can they help protect the body from the ongoing neurotoxic damage inflicted by lead or other toxic substances. Very often people will try supplementing with the depleted micronutrients—vitamin B_6 and magnesium being the most popular choices in this regard—and some short-term clinical benefit may be gained. Alas, these benefits are usually limited or short-lived, as once again the underlying cause has been overlooked.

The Neurotoxic Barrage: Harmful Chemicals

The mothers of autistic children often exhibit high levels of synthetic chemicals in their own bodies, which may then be passed on to their children during gestation or breastfeeding. Recent research indicates that those chemicals with lower molecular weights are more hazardous to the fetus, since they more rapidly enter the placenta. Such chemicals include some of the most common toxins found in our environment, such as carbon monoxide, polycyclic aromatic hydrocarbons, ethanol (alcohol), and PCBs.

Another danger is that many of these are lipophilic (fat-loving) compounds that can pass with relative ease through the skin of the fetus, which is not protected by the barriers it later develops. The chemicals then become concentrated in the fatty tissues of the fetus and, eventually, the newborn. The skin of a newborn is also highly absorptive since it has not yet keratinized (formed a tougher, keratin-rich covering), as this occurs during the first three to five days of life.[29] (A practical note: Parents should keep infants of any age away from areas that have been recently sprayed with pesticides, cleaned with toxic solvents, or exposed to any synthetic chemicals.)

A host of chemical exposures during gestation have been linked specifically to autism. Prenatal exposure to alcohol and drugs has been associated with autism.[30] Fetal alcohol syndrome and exposure to cocaine specifically have been associated with autism.[31] As I have mentioned, fetal exposure to thalidomide around days 20 to 24 after conception has been linked to autism.[32] The cause is thought to be a shortening of the brain stem, a defect that would occur during closure of the neural tube.[33]

Specifically, autism combined with moderate to severe mental retardation has also been linked to fetal alcohol exposure—though autistic behavior is not generally associated with prenatal exposure to alcohol.[34] In general, in utero alcohol exposure is associated with a range of neuropsy-chiatric disorders, including ADHD, Asperger's syndrome, and cognitive impairment.[35]

We should keep in mind here that many forms of toxic exposure during pregnancy have harmful effects on the fetus, though it is not yet clear if or how exactly they are linked to autism. Smoking marijuana during pregnancy definitely raises the risk of genotoxic effects on the fetus.[36] Tobacco smoke, too, is known to have such genotoxic effects.[37] Maternal smoking has been associated with impaired exhale "breathing" movements, or expelling of amniotic fluid from the lungs of the fetus.[38] And we have long known about the genotoxic effects of diethylstilbestrol, or DES, on the fetus,[39] which can lead to certain rare forms of cancer later in life.

Related research has shown that prenatal exposure to many hazardous chemicals, such as polycyclic aromatic hydrocarbons produced by liquefying coal, are also genotoxic. High levels of these chemicals have been shown to cause malformation of the fetus, growth retardation, and embryo lethality in mice; significant toxic potential for the fetus was noted even at low levels not considered toxic to the mother.[40] The fetus may also swallow amniotic fluid contaminated by xenobiotic chemicals that later disrupt the normal growth of flora in the intestinal tract.

Exposure to caffeine in utero may also interrupt abnormal neurological development in the fetus.[41] According to one theory, caffeine ingestion by the mother could lead to a disruption of rapid eye movement (REM) sleep of the fetus, which could lead to abnormal development of the brain. Caffeine also tends to tax the liver—and the defective liver would of course tend to amplify its toxic potential. Paradoxically, however, it can also be used to aid the later stages of detoxication.

PCBs are known to disrupt normal fetal development and to have consequences that may not manifest until later in life. In utero exposure to PCBs has been associated in at least one study with lower birth weight and head circumference, as well as other adverse effects, including memory deficits.[42] In Taiwan, children born to mothers who had eaten rice oil contaminated with a particularly toxic form of PCBs suffered a host of developmental abnormalities—physical, cognitive, and behavioral. PCBs have harmful effects on in vitro fertilization in mice, suppressing embryonic growth and having other toxic effects as well.[43] One disturbing set of studies indicated that PCB exposure in very early life can lead to abnormal development later on, during puberty.[44]

Some intriguing research also shows that the fetus's inability to metabolize certain substances may actually protect it from their toxic effects. For example, even if a pregnant woman has high acetaminophen levels, the fetus can't metabolize this chemical, so it is excreted, and the fetus's liver is not damaged by it.[45]

The mother's nutrition during pregnancy can also have a significant impact on the neurodevelopment of the fetus.[46] We know that nutrition during pregnancy influences the development of adult disease.[47] We don't yet know the mechanisms by which fetal diet affects risk of chronic disease—what periods of development are most vulnerable, or what type of malnutrition engenders what risks.

It is clear, however, that adequate levels of folate are crucial for normal fetal development. Folic acid plays an important role in reducing the risk of neural tube defects.[48] As I discussed in Chapter 3, some public health researchers have proposed that a high risk of neural tube defects may, in theory, translate into an increased risk of autism.[49] Inadequate levels of folate can also result in premature birth, which has been associated with a host of developmental disorders, including mental retardation, learning disabilities, and childhood psychiatric disorders.[50]

The recommended intake of folate for pregnant women is 600 micrograms daily.[51] We should also remember that fetal nutrition depends not only on the mother's nutritional intake during pregnancy, but also on the quality of her diet prior to conception.[52]

Reassembling the Puzzle of Autism

To recap, I've established in this chapter that some form of toxic injury triggers autism in very early life. A critical part of this injury is a fundamental weakening of the liver's detoxifying capacities. This abnormally functioning liver, in the context of ongoing exposure to toxins, leads to a scenario of toxic overload. This situation gives rise to the complex constellation of autistic symptoms.

All the clinical studies we have conducted give evidence supporting this scenario. Autistic children have elevated levels of neurotoxic chemicals and heavy metals in their bodies; at the same time, they exhibit an array of abnormal liver detoxication characteristics. In spite of the harmful effects of early toxic exposures, removing toxic substances from the bodies of these children leads to substantial improvements in autistic symptoms. As the body's systems are brought back into balance, these behaviors tend to subside. Over a period of twelve to thirty-six months of intense detoxication, chelation, and nutritional therapy, most of the children we have treated at the Edelson Center have shown significant improvement in autistic symptoms.

The fragility of the developing nervous system continues well into early life. An infant's interactions with the environment are particularly critical during the first several months of life, when neural connections are still forming. In fact, the infant's brain undergoes rapid growth and integration for the first few years of life.

Toxic and other forms of injury may therefore occur not only during gestation, but at birth or in infancy. Factors such as drugs consumed during pregnancy, a traumatic birth experience, and lack of breastfeeding in early life have all been shown to significantly impair early brain development. All three are associated with an average drop in IQ of 10 points or more.

Just as young brains need good food, they may also need social stimulation and parental "bonding" in order to grow properly. Some studies show that the infant's cognitive growth may depend heavily on mothering behaviors such as rocking, soothing, talking, or otherwise stimulating the young infant. For the child that can flip a switch, too much TV viewing may promote a passive orientation toward learning about the world. Jean Piaget, the Swiss psychologist who proposed a comprehensive theory of the development of intelligence, said a child's active exploration of the total environment is a prerequisite for normal intellectual growth.

If a child is born into the world with some degree of abnormal function, a diet and lifestyle that fail to promote normal brain activity will only exacerbate the handicap. Fortunately for us, the human brain is amazingly resilient. Prescriptive dietary changes and behavioral therapy can serve as a vehicle for healing the brain and nervous system. Even more fundamentally, though, an aggressive detoxification program can help stop the cycle of toxic overload, and allow the body's organ systems to regain normal functioning. With the right interventions—nutritional therapy, chelation of heavy metals, and targeted detoxification strategies—we can reverse this process.

Tim's story

Tim and his teacher Linda are sitting at a table in the classroom. "And these are . . . ?" she says, pointing to his ears. Tim, a slender, dark-haired boy of five, is rapidly chewing on a piece of gum. He looks at her but does not reply. "Your ears!" she says brightly, pointing to Tim's ears—"one, two." He turns his face to her, looks into her eyes, but it is as though he does not hear what she is saying.

"Let's color something you can hear with your ears," Linda suggests. "Would you like to color the bird singing, or the clock ringing, or the radio playing music, the lawnmower, or somebody reading you a story, or an airplane?" Tim does not answer.

Linda selects the picture of a radio playing music for Tim. "Okay, now pick a crayon. Would you color this picture, please?" Silently, Tim reaches out and takes five or six crayons from the box.

"Tim, please pick one crayon," Linda says patiently. "Which one are you going to use? Pick one color." Tim looks down at the crayons, hands one crayon to Linda, and clutches the rest in his hand.

"Color this for me," she says. Tim looks at her, puts the crayons down, then holds his index finger rigidly against the page as though pointing at the picture. He glances quizzically at Linda. Finally she puts a crayon in his hand and puts the crayon to the paper. He begins to color, but he colors randomly, outside the lines, as though the picture were not even there.

Tim was born in September 1989. At first, everything seemed normal. His parents were delighted when he spoke his first words. But a few months later, a disturbing change began to take place. Shortly after Tim began to talk, he gradually stopped using the new words he had learned. By the time he was twenty months old, he had stopped talking entirely. He became withdrawn and tearful, avoided being touched, and cried for hours for no apparent reason. Alarmed, his parents took him to several specialists, trying to determine the cause of these changes.

Tim was not formally diagnosed with autism until age three and a half. At that time, he began a program of nutritional therapy. In November 1995, when he was six, he underwent three months of steroid treatment, and showed mild improvement. He also underwent auditory integration training and speech therapy.

Tim's parents first brought him to my office in April 1996, when he was seven years old. Tim's mother explained that although he had shown some slight improvement from the treatments he had received, he was still distant, easily frustrated, caught in the grip of classic autistic behavioral symptoms.

As Tim sat in my office, I could see this for myself. He made low grunting sounds, his eyes scanned the room, and he often squinted nervously, as though the light in my office was too bright for him.

Later, when I examined Tim, I discovered that in fact he suffered from abnormal sensitivity to light and sound. This was part of a whole pattern of symptoms that together formed a picture of classic autism. He squinted habitually, and although he was capable of simple speech, he often communicated in guttural sounds instead. Tim also exhibited delayed echolalia, or echoing of others' speech. If he spoke at all, he spoke rapidly, reversed pronouns, and frequently dropped consonants.

Tim's parents told me that he was often destructive, pushed people away, had a short attention span, and suffered from insomnia. At home he spent much of his time climbing furniture obsessively. He was withdrawn, unable to reason, and had difficulty learning. He suffered from constant anxiety and mood swings. He had frequent screaming tantrums, especially when his demands were not met immediately, and attempts at discipline had little effect on his behavior.

After performing a thorough physical examination, and taking a detailed medical history from Tim's parents, we ran several tests to ascertain the level of toxins and heavy metals in Tim's system. These tests provided important information for our treatment of Tim. Tests showed he had high levels of tin, lead, tolulene (greater than 1,000 percent of the amount considered safe for adults), and trimethylbenzene (150 percent of the adult maximum). He showed certain autoimmune characteristics, including Purkinje cell antibodies and myelin basic protein antibody. We also found that Tim had renal loss of the key neurotransmitters epinephrine and dopamine. He also suffered from nutritional and pancreatic deficiencies, maldigestion, malabsorption, abnormal liver detoxication (partly reflected in elevated mercapturic acid levels).

Even though we were beginning treatment with Tim relatively late, at age seven, I felt confident that I could help him. At the very least, we had to rid his body of the toxic burden with which he was struggling. I put Tim on a long-term regimen of nutritional therapy and detoxication. His treatments included EDTA therapy to remove heavy metals, sauna therapy to remove chemicals, nutritional therapy and liver upregulation controlled with nutrition, environmental controls, an avoidance diet, enzyme therapies for maldigestion, and glutamine and aloe vera for gastrointestinal tract maintenance.

Within one year, Tim showed an estimated improvement of 80 percent across the board. He showed dramatic improvement in social and cognitive abilities, and his autistic behaviors, such as squinting and throwing tantrums, appeared now only occasionally. It was as though he was making up for lost time, learning new vocabulary words, excelling in math and reading comprehension tests.

Linda, Tim's teacher, was astounded by his progress during this period. Linda and I talked with Tim one day about a year after he began treatment with me.

"Where do you live?" she asks him.

"Cleveland, Ohio."

"That's right! And what is your address?"

Tim gives his address correctly. He answers several other questions—he has a brother, he is in second grade, he is eight years old.

Whatever world Tim inhabited before, it is as though he is back now, a shy newcomer among his classmates and teachers. He talks in a faltering, quiet voice, but responds and communicates in a way that would have been unthinkable a year ago.

Linda asks Tim a series of mathematical questions. How much money is two nickels and two pennies?

"Twelve cents," he says slowly.

"Twelve cents, that's right!" She holds up her hand and he gives her a high-five.

"Okay," Linda says, holding out a yo-yo, "this yo-yo is twenty-five cents for the quarter, five cents for the nickel. How much money does it cost in all?"

"Thirty cents."

"Right, thirty cents!" Another high-five. "A cupcake is a dime, a nickel, and two pennies. How much money?"

"Seventeen cents." Tim speaks quietly but clearly, thinking over the answer for a moment before he speaks.

"Seventeen cents! You got them all right!" Delighted, his teacher exchanges high-fives with him again, and he smiles shyly.

Chapter 7

◆

In-Depth Diagnosis: A Key to Effective Therapy

When three-year-old Bruce Johnson was diagnosed with autism, an amazing act of humanity occurred. Family, friends, residents, and businesses in Bruce's home town of Royston, Canada, together raised $29,000 to pay for him and his family to travel to our Atlanta clinic for diagnostic testing and treatment.

At the Edelson Center, the first thing we did was to take a detailed environmental and family history of the Johnsons, including medical histories for Bruce and both his parents. Next I performed a thorough physical examination on Bruce. Finally, we did a series of important laboratory tests designed to measure Bruce's liver detoxication, digestive and immune functions, and the presence of toxic chemicals and heavy metals in his body.

When the test results came back a few weeks later, they revealed a pattern that by now was all too familiar to me. Yet I knew that it meant we would be able to help Bruce recover. The tests showed that Bruce's liver was unable to effectively detoxify wastes and environmental toxins. In Bruce's body we found nearly nine times the adult average level of the petrochemical xylene, as well as three times the average level of benzene. Bruce also had high levels of lead. He suffered from nutritional deficiencies, malabsorption and maldigestion, and allergies to a number of foods, chemicals, and molds.

For many, the battery of tests we ran on Bruce may seem prohibitively expensive. Without these tests, however, Bruce's syndrome of toxic exposure, the underlying cause of his autistic symptoms, would never have come to light. These laboratory tests, along with a detailed medical history and physical examination, form the core of our diagnostic program. They are the first essential step to improving this illness, the starting point from which we go on to develop an individualized treatment program suited to the needs of each autistic child we treat.

Bruce was fortunate that his community rallied around him and raised the funds to make his diagnosis and treatment process possible. He received a month of treatment at our center, including a detoxification program of daily saunas, chelation to remove heavy metals from the body, exercise, and intensive nutritional therapy.

In Bruce's case, the timing of his visit to our center was also ideal. Three years old may be early enough to successfully treat and possibly reverse many if not all of the symptoms of autism. Nevertheless, once we have performed these diagnostic tests, the efficacy of the therapy is never guaranteed. A lot depends on the age of the child when we begin treatment. The older the child, the more difficult the job of reversing the process is. Most of the children who come to me for treatment are already older than Bruce, yet we have witnessed some amazing recoveries and reversals of disease.

At our Atlanta center, the comprehensive treatment program we recommend for autistic children is demanding. This program lasts an average 19.8 months. In the beginning, both parents and children must devote themselves for weeks at a time to daily saunas, taking many nutritional supplements, and chelation therapy, all of which can be difficult, uncomfortable, and time-consuming. No matter which course of therapy we decide on for each individual child, we also encourage children and families to continue participating in behavioral modification programs to stimulate dendritic and neuronal development. All of this requires of both parents and children a great deal of patience and perseverance.

This program is also, however, immensely effective and rewarding. According to parental evaluations using the ATEC questionnaire (described later in this chapter), the average stated improvement in our patients after approximately two years of treatment is 67.5 percent. Many parents are astonished at how rapidly their children begin to make progress in developing verbal and social skills once they begin the detoxification process.

I have been studying the biology of the autistic illnesses for the past decade. At the beginning of this journey, the various parameters that reflect the characteristics of this syndrome were, for me, still mostly theoretical. Today, after studying nearly 200 children in a very comprehensive way, I feel confident in saying that the testing I am about to describe allows me to form a complete understanding of the biology of this illness, and makes possible the improvement and possible reversal of this illness.

In this chapter I will explain the diagnostic tests we perform, why we do them, and how each one contributes to a complete picture of autistic illness in each child, a picture that is different for every individual.

Why Lab Testing Matters

At the Edelson Center, we perform a range of tests to gauge the level and type of toxic burden in each autistic child that we treat. Most of the children we see have already been diagnosed with some form of autistic spectrum disorder. I am less interested in the fine points of naming this disease, and more concerned with getting at the root *cause* of the autistic behavior in each individual child.

Many parents of my autistic patients have expressed concern at how expensive these laboratory tests can be. Parents often want to know how necessary these tests really are. This is not the typical laboratory work that most physicians perform. Because of its sophisticated and labor-intensive nature, labs tend to charge higher fees for these tests. This is a time-consuming and expensive proposition, but it is necessary if we are to treat the cause, rather than the symptoms, of this illness.

The most important tests we perform include the following: (1) an amino acid analysis to measure digestion, absorption, and nutritional deficiencies; (2) a heavy metal challenge to identify the number, type, and amount of heavy metals present; (3) skin testing to determine which allergies are present; (4) blood testing for xenobiotic chemicals such as hydrocarbons, organophosphates, and chlorinated pesticides; (5) a liver detoxication profile showing how well the phase I and phase II processes of liver detoxication are functioning; (6) antibody studies to measure autoimmunity, specifically the immune response to the brain. Because autism is an illness that involves multiple organ systems, it is crucial that we understand which systems are functioning adequately and which are impaired so that we can tailor our treatment program accordingly; (7) peptide study to look at gluten and casein levels; (8) IqA sensitivity to gluten and casein; (9) stool study for abnormal ecology of the gastrointestinal tract; (10) mineral levels; (11) other miscellaneous studies.

I understand autism to be a neurotoxic syndrome, which poses special problems when we try to identify the nature of the toxic exposure through laboratory tests. First, we use these lab tests to determine the levels of toxins in the bodies of our autistic patients; but this is deceiving because blood levels reflect probably only one hundredth of levels of xenobiotic chemicals stored in body fat. Second, often the neurotoxic damage has occurred in utero or early life, and the neurotoxins that have inflicted the damage are already long gone from the body. Low-level chronic exposure can also play a large role, however, in the etiology of autism. Testing for the presence of toxins and their effects on the organ systems of the body is necessary because it can give us information about what kind of neurotoxic damage has occurred, or is occurring.

Neurotoxic disease is also difficult to diagnose because its effects on the central nervous system are usually systemic, rather than localized. Neurotoxins tend to cause cell death, myelin dysfunction, and degeneration of axons throughout the nervous system.[1] To further complicate matters, various levels of exposure to a single toxin may trigger different sets of symptoms; and exposure to one neurotoxin can exacerbate the effects of another that might otherwise remain relatively harmless.[2]

All of this presents a highly complex picture to be sorted out, and before we begin any laboratory testing, we make use of two other important diagnostic tools—the physical examination and the medical history. The physical examination is valuable because it may reveal subtle symptoms that may have gone unnoticed, and because it gives me an immediate sense of the overall state of the child's health.

Lastly, I always take a detailed medical history of not only the autistic child, but the whole family. This is important for pinpointing the scope and timing of any possible toxic exposure. A parent with an occupation that involves chemical exposure, recent home renovations or pesticide sprays, lead paint, the number of silver amalgams in the mother and grandmother—all of these are red flags, crucial clues that shed light on this neurotoxic phenomenon and how it is being manifested in the child.

Chemical Toxicity Blood Levels

Over 97 percent of the autistic children I have treated are burdened with very high levels of xenobiotics, or toxic environmental chemicals. One of the most important tests that we perform measures the blood levels of these chemicals. These chemicals live in the fatty tissues of the body.

Since the brain is about 70 percent fat, this is one of the first places to which the chemicals migrate. In fetal and postnatal life, there is no protective blood-brain barrier in place, so it is easy for these chemicals to enter the brain and interfere with brain function at the most vulnerable stage of development.

As I have mentioned, the blood levels of these chemicals are only about one hundredth of the levels stored in the body's fat tissues. Ideally, we would evaluate levels of these chemicals in the fat tissues, but this is not practical since it would mean having to do multiple fat biopsies. We therefore have to be satisfied with a less than perfect study. We can improve the accuracy of the results of this test by having the patient spend two hours in the sauna (over an eight-hour period) at 160 degrees. However, this again is quite impractical.

The most common chemicals that we find in this test are the aromatic hydrocarbons—benzene, xylene, and toluene. The next most common are the organophosphates, and chlorinated pesticides are the third most common chemicals that come up in this test.

As we have seen, all of these chemicals are found in our environment. Some of the most common sources include paints, gasoline, carpets, inks, adhesives, pesticides, herbicides, detergents, insecticides, polishes, cleaning solvents, cigarette smoke, pharmaceuticals, perfumes, dyes, rubber, Styrofoam, dry-cleaning chemicals, photo-processing chemicals, plastics, and rubber.

It is vitally important to measure the toxic burden in each patient so that we can understand exactly which substances need to be removed, as well as the baseline levels, so that later we can measure the results of treatment.

Heavy Metal Evaluation

Heavy metals are a group of toxic metals found in our environment. I have observed that autistic patients often have a massive burden of these metals in their tissues. The heavy metals include mercury, tin, lead, cadmium, nickel, aluminum, arsenic, and antimony. The most common of these are mercury, tin, and lead, which are also those we most often find to be elevated in our autistic patients.

It is very important to understand that these metals are stored in the tissues of the body. They spend only a very short time in the blood. They are not usually found in the blood or urine, unless there has been a recent exposure or there is such a high level in the body that it spills into the blood, and therefore into the urine. Note that heavy metal toxicity will vary from one individual to the next. These individual differences in response to heavy metals are probably due to two factors: (1) genetic factors that influence the availability of the sulfur-containing compounds, glutathione and metallothionein, which in turn modify the distribution and toxicity of certain metals; and (2) deficiencies of specific nutrients, which in turn can modify the excretion and toxicity of certain metals.

Thus when a physician takes a blood sample from a child and says there is no sign of any heavy metal in the body, he is not giving you accurate or comprehensive information. He can only state with certainty that there is no sign of any toxic metal in the blood at the time he has tested the blood.

The gold standard technique for determining the levels of heavy metals in the body is to give the patient chelators that bind to the metals in the tissues and pull them into the urine, which is then tested within twelve to twenty-four hours. Only this type of "heavy metal challenge" can give accurate results. In addition, we also use hair analysis to provide supplementary information about the heavy metal burden.

Liver Detoxication Study

Until now, the underlying role of the liver has been overlooked in autism. The most common liver defect is an overactive phase I detoxication system. The second most common defect is impaired sulfoxidation, and the ability to produce the sulfate molecule, which is needed for part of phase II detoxication.

Why is it necessary to perform this study if we already know that nearly all autistic children have these problems? The answer is that we can never be sure exactly which part of the liver's detoxication system is working inefficiently, and only when we know this can the proper nutritional upregulation be devised to improve the function. This test is done by swallowing aspirin, Tylenol, and caffeine, and then collecting urine, saliva, and blood to measure the presence of various compounds that give us information about these functions.

Amino Acid Analysis

The amino acid analysis is a vital part of the evaluation of children with autistic spectrum disorders. In my clinical experience with over a hundred amino acid analyses in these children, it is unusual to find a child who doesn't have biochemical abnormalities that can be elucidated with the use of this tool. These abnormalities may include malabsorption, maldigestion, amino acid deficiencies, vitamin and mineral deficiencies, abnormal levels of stomach acid, and other factors. As mentioned earlier, we have found a syndrome of malabsorption in more than 50 percent of these children.

The most accurate way to evaluate the amino acid biochemistry is to do a 24-hour urine collection, making sure that the child drinks plenty of fluids and that each meal contains plenty of protein. Because we don't want to lose any of the urine for this test, in some cases it may be necessary to catheterize a child in order to be sure that the collection is complete.

Intestinal Permeability

The intestinal permeability test allows us to determine whether a child is suffering from either intestinal malabsorption or "leaky gut" syndrome. Both of these intestinal abnormalities have been found in a high percentage of autistic children. My clinical observations suggest that these abnormalities contribute not only to digestive problems, but also to immune and inflammatory imbalances in the body. This test involves drinking a liquid containing the compounds lactulose and mannitol, and then collecting urine later for a specific period of time. The results give us information about whether the intestinal membrane is functioning normally.

Biochemical Profile

A child's overall biochemical status has a great deal to do with his or her behavior and overall functioning. This is a general evaluation that measures the following functions, which are all related to some form of internal injury: cellular blood count, liver enzyme tests, calcium and phosphorus metabolism, electrolyte balance, lipid metabolism, thyroid metabolism, ferritin (iron storage), protein, albumin, and globulin chemistry, kidney function, and sugar metabolism.

Allergy Testing

Every autistic child we have tested has allergies. These allergies are often "delayed" and may not always show up as obvious allergic manifestations such as a runny nose, skin rash, asthma, watery eyes, and other classic symptoms. These delayed reactions may not show up for hours after the offending allergen enters the body. Some symptoms of delayed type allergy may include: hyperactivity, colitis, migraine headaches, abdominal pain, eczema, tinnitus, fibromyalgia, tachycardia, bed wetting, and many others.

Once we pinpoint the substances to which a child is allergic, we can develop a protocol for avoiding those substances, which can substantially reduce both behavioral and physiological symptom—symptoms that often parents have not even previously thought were connected to exposure to these allergens.

Another allergy study, the IgG blood test, is somewhat controversial. There is a lot of debate about whether a positive result for this test can be directly correlated to allergic symptoms.

Blood Cell Mineral Levels

This blood test shows levels of various minerals in the body. About 90% of the autistic children I have treated have suffered from major mineral deficiencies. The most common deficiencies are zinc, magnesium, potassium, and selenium. It is vital to know which of these has to be increased, so the cellular function can be made more efficient.

Functional Vitamin Levels

Measuring concentrations of specific vitamins can give us a clearer idea of which micronutrient deficits require the most aggressive attention. Nontheless, this blood test is not among the routine evaluations we use. Whether we use it or not depends on how extreme the autistic problems are in a particular patient, and whether I feel I can use my clinical judgment to give the patient the proper nutrients without this test being done.

Gliadin and Casein IgA Evaluation

This is a simple blood test for antibodies to two proteins called gliadin and casein. Some autistic children form antibodies to these two proteins. It is very important to know whether this is the case—so we can remove foods containing these proteins from the patient's diet.

Comprehensive Stool Analysis

As I noted above, many autistic children have problems related to the gastrointestinal tract. They may have intestinal overgrowths of bacteria, fungi, or parasites that can cause abnormal immune function. From this analysis, we can tell a lot about the health of the gastrointestinal tract, including its absorption, digestion, immune system, and whether or not the normal ecology of this system has been disrupted. This is an easy test to do, requiring only a stool sample collection.

Neuroimmunotoxicological Study

This diagnostic procedure reveals the complex interrelationship of a dysregulated immune system and the nervous system. It measures blood antibodies that attack protein fragments in the central nervous system. These protein fragments may include myelin basic protein, neuronal antibodies, glial fibrillary acid protein, and others. If antibodies to any of these are found, the treatment of choice is usually to use megadoses of gamma globulin to stop the immune system from attacking the nervous system. We also use transfer factor and oral myelin desensitization to provide additional information about the immune-CNS interaction.

Immune System Evaluation

Depending on the individual patient and the history of infectious disease or other unusual abnormal immune symptoms, we may also consider performing immune-related studies such as natural killer cell function, immunoglobulin profiles, mitogen stimulation studies, or phagocytic index. Some studies have also indicated that this group has elevated levels of IL-12 and gamma interferon.

Organic Acid Analysis

In most patients we recommend this test. It enables us to assess various aspects of intermediary biochemistry, the molecular workings of cell functions. This test also provides information about vitamins, minerals, trace elements, amino acids, and organic acids. We don't run this test routinely. This test requires collection of the first voided specimen of urine in the morning.

Temporal Brain Cortex (Endothelial Capillary) Autoantibody Study

This is a relatively new test that was developed at Washington University in St. Louis. The test is a measure of the antibodies in the blood of the patient that attack the endothelial lining in the temporal cortex of the brain. The published study showed that 36 percent of autistic children had positive antibodies to the cortex. We have done about fifteen of these studies on autistic children, and found six patients who tested positive for these antibodies.

Neurotransmitter Study

This method enables us to measure the levels of certain key neurotransmitters, including serotonin, epinephrine, and dopamine, in the patient's urine and blood platelets. The test is optional and can be helpful in a comprehensive evaluation of the neurochemistry of the patient. It is both a blood and urine study.

Essential Fatty Acid Analysis

We use this blood analysis to evaluate the patient's fatty acid metabolism. Again, this is an optional test but can be very useful in adding to our knowledge of the patient's biochemistry.

Measuring Results: The ATEC Questionnaire

We use another important diagnostic tool both prior to and after completion of treatment at our clinic. This is the Autistic Treatment Evaluation Checklist (ATEC), a detailed checklist developed by the Autism Research Institute. This questionnaire, which is usually completed by the parents, is very important for testing the effectiveness of treatment.

We use this checklist to numerically calculate the status of specific autistic characteristics in our patients, by comparing scores prior to and following treatment. A simple scoring procedure calculates subscale scores and an overall summary score for the ATEC. Scores are weighted according to the response and corresponding subscale. The higher the subscale and total scores, the more impaired the subject.

Figure 7-1

ATEC

Here is the ATEC checklist created by the Autism Research Institute that we use to evaluate the effectiveness of our treatment protocol for autistic children. This checklist is divided into four types of symptoms: (I) Speech/Language/ Communication; (II) Sociability; (III) Sensory/Cognitive Awareness; (IV) and Health/ Physical/ Behavior. The questionnaire first asks for the assessment period, official diagnosis of the child, and personal details such as sex and date of birth.

I—Speech/Language/Communication

N=not true, S=somewhat true, or V=very true

---

knows own name
responds to "no" or "stop"
can follow some commands
can use one word at a time
can use 2 words at a time
can use 3 words at a time
knows 10 or more words
can use sentences with 4 or more words
explains what he/she wants
asks meaningful questions
speech tends to be meaningful/relevant
often uses several successive sentences
carries on fairly good conversation
has normal ability to communicate for his/her age

II—Sociability

N=not descriptive, S=somewhat descriptive, V=very descriptive

---

seems to be in a shell—you cannot reach him/her
ignores other people
pays little or no attention when addressed
uncooperative and resistant
no eye contact
prefers to be left alone
shows no affection
fails to greet parents
avoids contact with others

does not imitate
dislikes being held/cuddled
does not share or show
does not wave "bye bye"
disagreeable/not compliant
temper tantrums
lacks friends/companions
rarely smiles
insensitive to others' feelings
indifferent to being liked
indifferent if parent(s) leave

III—Sensory/Cognitive Awareness

N=not descriptive, S=somewhat descriptive, V=very descriptive

---

responds to own name
responds to praise
looks at people and animals
looks at pictures (and TV)
does drawing, coloring, art
plays with toys appropriately
appropriate facial expression
understands stories on TV
understands explanations
aware of environment
aware of danger
shows imagination
initiates activities
dresses self
curious, interested
venturesome—explores
"tuned in"—not spacey
looks where others are looking

IV—Health/Physical/Behavior

N=not a problem, MI=minor problem, MO=moderate problem, S=serious problem

bed-wetting
wets pants/diapers
soils pants/diapers
diarrhea
constipation

sleep problems
eats too much/too little
extremely limited diet
hyperactive
lethargic
hits or injures self
hits or injures others
destructive
sound-sensitive
anxious/fearful
unhappy/crying
seizures
obsessive speech
rigid routines
shouts or screams
demands sameness
often agitated
not sensitive to pain
"hooked" or fixated on certain objects/topics
repetitive movements

Note: The Autism Treatment Evaluation Checklist (ATEC) was developed by Bernard Rimland, Ph.D. and Stephen Edelson, Ph.D. of the Autism Research Institute and is used here by permission of its authors.

Nigel's Story

Nigel Aujero gazed calmly at me as he sat on his father's lap in my office. Unlike many of the autistic children I have treated, he was not fidgety and did not flap his hands or glance around the room. He sat quietly watching our faces and listening to our conversation.

The Aujeros had arrived the night before from Italy. They had decided to bring their son, Nigel, age six and a half, to see me in Atlanta after hearing about our program from another family. Nigel's father, Armond, was slight and sandy-haired, with glasses, and a slightly mirthful manner. He was a professor of computer science at a university in Rome. Nigel's mother, Regina, sat quietly, with the same still, fragile air as her son, who had her soft brown eyes and dark hair.

Nigel's parents, like their son, also struck me as different from many of the other families of autistic children that I'd met. They did not seem over-whelmed or discouraged, with that look of burned-out exhaustion that I had seen in so many parents' faces, but only single-mindedly determined to help their son.

"Tell me about Nigel," I said, returning the boy's gaze. He did not take his eyes from mine. He looked pale and fragile in his father's arms. "When was he first diagnosed with autism?"

"Nigel was okay until he was about fourteen months old," his father told me. The problems began, he said, a few months after Nigel received his MMR shot.

"Within a few months we started to see regression, Dr. Edelson. Before he was two years old I felt that something was really wrong. It was another year before a professional felt unafraid enough to give us the diagnosis. When he was three, a neuropsychologist diagnosed Nigel with PDD with autistic features. But by the time he was two, I already knew something was completely wrong."

I asked what he meant by regression. What were the signs that had led them to suspect that something was wrong?

The biggest sign, said Armond, was that Nigel's newly acquired lan-guage abilities began to disappear. "Nigel was talking before, even in sets of two words, like 'open door,' or 'open sweets,'" he told me. "And then a few months after the shot, he disappeared completely. He became—I can-not say autistic, because it was not the first thing that came to my mind at that time—but I saw regression in his speech and behavior. He started to cry a lot, throw tantrums, and push us away. He showed all the signs that we can now understand were PDD."

The actual diagnosis, however, hit Armond and Regina with devastat-ing force. They heard the word "autism" and pictured their son living out his life alone in an institution. They spent a week crying together, mourn-ing for their son. "Then we decided to fight," Armond told me. "We de-cided not to lose any time."

Right away Armond and Regina began researching treatments for their son. They took Nigel to see many doctors and therapists—psychologists, pediatric neurologists, behavioral specialists, speech therapists. They started their son on an intensive behavioral modification program, com-bined with sensory integration therapy to help improve his ability to pro-cess auditory and visual stimuli. But he was not improving very quickly. There were only tiny glimmers of possibility, followed by long discourag-ing periods when he did not improve much, so they kept searching.

When Nigel was six, Armond and Regina heard about our clinic from another family whose son had been treated here. They contacted us and arranged to bring their son to the clinic.

I told Armond and Regina that I suspected that Nigel, like so many of the autistic children I had treated, was suffering from a syndrome of some kind of toxicity. We just had to find out what kind—that would point the way to the right combination of therapies for him. Inwardly I felt thankful that Armond and Regina already knew how much this program would demand of them, and of Nigel. They were familiar already with the expensive battery of tests that would be necessary to pinpoint Nigel's individual toxic injuries, as well as his liver, gastrointestinal tract, and immune function abnormalities.

I explained the program to them in detail anyway, and they nodded as I spoke. We would test Nigel for allergies, as well as liver function, digestion, and the presence of various toxic chemicals and heavy metals in his body.

"You've come to the right place," I said, hoping not to raise their hopes too much, but feeling a determined sense, on some level, that I would be able to help Nigel.

"If we start now," I said, "I think there is a good chance that Nigel will regain a great deal of his cognitive abilities. If you can do only one thing for your son now, we should start here—not trying to modify his behavior, but focusing on the underlying physical cause of his illness. I can't promise you anything, but this is the fastest way I know for us to help your son."

"We trust you, Dr. Edelson," Armond said, looking down at Nigel, who was now asleep in his arms. "We have seen what you did for our friend's son. We're ready to do whatever is necessary. And we want to start right away."

That attitude proved to be the Aujero family's most valuable asset in their quest to help their son.

We began right away. The next morning, after taking a detailed medical history and doing a thorough physical examination, we performed a series of laboratory tests on Nigel, to measure his liver detoxication, levels of toxins, and other factors.

A few weeks later, Nigel's test results confirmed what I had suspected. The test results showed that Nigel suffered from food allergies, maldigestion, pancreatic insufficiency, and abnormal liver detoxication. He also had an overgrowth of harmful organisms in his gastrointestinal tract—including candidiasis, pseudomnas, giardia. Significantly, we found elevated levels of tin, lead, mercury, and several toxic chemicals. We also found that he was suffering from deficiencies of magnesium and zinc. It was a pattern I recognized immediately. Although Nigel's levels of heavy metals were elevated to abnormal levels, this was also a good sign, because it meant that chelation therapy would likely have significant therapeutic effects.

It turned out that the Aujeros meant what they said at the beginning. They were in this for the long haul. They wanted to begin detoxification treatment at the clinic right away, and they were prepared to stay in Atlanta for as long as necessary.

It was October 1997 when we began Nigel's treatment.

The Aujeros spent the next month and a half going through the detoxification program at the clinic, which involved daily saunas, chelation, nutritional therapy, and supplements. A few months later they would repeat this program, returning to Atlanta for another six-week round of detoxification.

Throughout the treatments, Nigel behaved calmly, never fighting or resisting going into the sauna, taking his many supplements or going on the treadmill, as other children often did. It was almost as though he knew, on some level, that all of this would help him.

"We are lucky to have a child whom we could make understand that this was for his own good," Armond told me quietly after the first course of detoxification. "He was really cooperative."

"Even though he is only six and a half, it was amazing," he went on. "We were constantly amazed that a child so young could do this. I cannot say it was difficult for us, because Nigel was not showing signs of distress, saying, 'Oh, this is tough, help me, help me!' When we come to your office, he pulls open the door himself, and he seems really happy. Even now, months later, we have an agreement—when he touches something that he shouldn't, I say 'Remember, Dr. Edelson doesn't like that,' and he respects that."

Nigel's parents noticed striking changes in Nigel's behavior almost immediately after beginning the detoxification program. First they noticed that he began to make more eye contact than he ever had before. Then his tantrums, in which he would alternately laugh and cry, completely stopped. These changes did not surprise me, since I knew we were on the right track in our treatment of Nigel. It was clearer to me than ever that autism had its roots in a syndrome of toxic injury that usually goes undiagnosed in autistic children.

After that first round of detoxification, Nigel's parents also reported that his quantitative skills were changing. Before coming to the Edelson Center, Nigel could answer questions about math only if the question was written down or counted on the fingers. Over the first course of detoxification, however, Nigel became more and more skilled in math. His parents were astonished, as much by his improvement as by the fact that, for a while, his abilities seemed to fluctuate almost from day to day. One moment he would be unable to answer simple math questions, then for the next twenty minutes he could suddenly answer a whole series of more difficult questions.

As the detoxification process continued, Nigel's abilities in true math began to surface. As the treatment progressed, their child's intelligence began to emerge. By the time a year had passed, these changes had taken root. By then, any question of whether or not Nigel was intelligent had disappeared.

Both Regina and Armond reported to me that they noticed a great change in their son after detoxification, especially after chelation therapy to remove heavy metals from his body. Allergies also played a crucial role. What produced these results was not a single factor, but a comprehensive approach that took the unique characteristics of Nigel's illness into account.

After a year and a half of the treatment, combined with behavioral therapies, no one could deny that the change in Nigel was immense. Family friends began remarking on how different he was.

Regina and Armond said that in the years of behavioral therapy Nigel had done before he came to me, he had never improved this rapidly. It had always been slow, uncertain progress.

"We put a lot of effort into behavioral treatments for Nigel," Regina said. "He was going to therapy with horses and swimming, sensory integration therapy, speech therapy. He was moving forward, but it was really one step at a time. You had to wait one year to see some changes, and still it was really one step. We saw the first big changes after a year and a half of your treating Nigel."

"We started to gain a child," Armond added. "The child with all his potential started to come out."

The Aujeros returned to our clinic several times over the next couple of years for Nigel's checkups. After the two initial six-week detoxification treatments, Nigel stayed on the treatment program for three years. His parents maintained a strict gluten- and casein-free diet, and kept his allergies under control. Every morning he took handfuls of vitamins and nutritional supplements.

After three years, the Aujeros cut back on some of these supplements, though they retained the core of vitamins, amino acids, and antioxidants that I had prescribed. The family purchased a sauna, and they continue with sauna therapy, not every day but on a regular basis. Nigel is still undergoing sensory integration therapy to improve his processing of visual and auditory data. Today, Nigel's therapeutic activities include riding horses and playing basketball with his peers—something his parents would never have imagined possible three years ago.

Over a period of forty-two months, Nigel exhibited an approximately 90 percent improvement in autistic symptoms, based on our clinical assessments. His parents report that he is improving all the time. The changes are evident from week to week. His sense of humor is developing, and he communicates more effectively, in a way that is almost caught up with that of his peers. He is now ten and a half, and his father says his communication skills are rapidly closing the age gap—he now talks and plays like a nine-year-old.

Nigel's math skills have also continued to improve. He has become a gifted math student. "He's really a 'math mind,' " his father told me proudly. "He's amazing, even for his age group. He's at the top of his class."

Chapter 8

◆

Nutritional Medicine to Support Your Child's Recovery

The human brain needs sound nutrition for normal functioning. This commonsense precept carries even greater significance when it comes to the brains of young children. We've known for decades that a child's daily diet exerts a profound influence over his thinking, behavior, and experience. A wealth of research has identified powerful links between food factors and mental factors. As my own clinical observations attest, this is vital information for the treatment of autistic children.

Autistic children frequently exhibit deficiencies in certain nutrients that are considered vital for proper brain function. Prominent among these deficiencies are trace elements such as magnesium, iron, copper, and zinc. But the impact of nutrition for the autistic child extends far beyond the brain itself. A poor diet can worsen the vicious cycle of malabsorption, maldigestion, impaired immune function, and abnormal liver detoxication that I have seen in all the autistic children coming through my Atlanta clinic.

Getting the right nutrients to help correct these imbalances can be a formidable challenge, as many of the parents I've worked with have come to realize. Because autistic children are notoriously "picky eaters," diet alone is unlikely to provide enough of each therapeutic nutrient needed to correct the biological imbalances found in autism.

My program incorporates an individually tailored nutritional program for each patient. The goal is to select a combination of foods and supplements that bolster the body's innate ability to heal itself. We also eliminate foods that may be potential allergic triggers, an aspect of diet that I will address in the next chapter. It is often challenging for parents to get their children to take the many nutritional supplements I prescribe, but this is a cornerstone of our program. We must strengthen the body—support healthy brain function, enhance immune function, and improve digestion and detoxication. Proper nutrition can help awaken the body's own innate forces of health and balance, helping to break this cycle.

Feeding the Brain and Whole Body

Our nutritional program focuses mainly on a regimen of nutritional supplements and therapeutic diets to treat food allergies. In addition, we encourage parents to adhere to the principles of optimal nutrition. This means keeping their children on a healthy, diet centered around organically grown whole grains, fruits, and vegetables. Diet has a direct influence on brain function, and a junk-food diet of foods high in fat and sugar can undermine the most vigilant program of detoxification for an autistic patient. A healthy diet is vital for shoring up the body's own defenses against toxic injury, strengthening the nervous, digestive, and immune systems. The right nutritional balance is vital for achieving normal brain function, and can have an enormous impact on memory, cognition, and basic intelligence.

It's hard to imagine that just a decade ago, most scientists viewed the brain as relatively impervious to the vagaries of dietary change. The blood-brain barrier was thought to protect the brain from dramatic changes in blood chemistry caused by diet and drug abuse. Only under extreme conditions, such as lead or mercury poisoning, could blood-borne "insults" to the brain result in serious problems. This view, however, is now known to be incomplete, particularly where young children are concerned. The latest research indicates that specific nutrients and nutrient combinations can enhance problem-solving ability, heighten alertness and attention span, and improve mood and behavior in normal children. Other elements or food factors, in contrast, can exacerbate behavioral problems in children who are already impaired by neurodevelopmental deficits; these factors further limit their efforts to process information and interact with their world.

C. Keith Connors, Ph.D., director of Duke University's Center for Attention Deficit Disorders in Children and author of *Feeding the Brain: How Foods Affect Children* (Plenum Press, 1989) has identified many important relations between food and a child's behavior and "intelligence quotient" or I.Q.[1] Another pioneering researcher who has helped shape our understanding of diet's effects on the mind is Judith Wurtman, Ph.D., a research scientist at the Massachusetts Institute of Technology and author of *Managing Your Mind and Mood Through Food* (Rawson Associates, 1986). According to Dr. Wurtman, the mood mechanisms of the brain are finely tuned, and even small, short-term chemical changes can markedly influence the way a person feels, thinks, and performs. Even a single meal can alter one's ability to think, learn, and communicate effectively with others.[2] For both Connors and Wurtman, then, food, mind, and mood are inextricably linked, and the impact of diet on brain function has been underestimated.

A landmark contribution to the study of nutritional influences on the mind was the 340-page report, *Nutrition and Mental Health,* sponsored by the U.S. Senate Select Committee on Nutrition and Human Needs in 1980. This report documents links between various nutrient deficiencies—notably zinc, magnesium, iron, and vitamins B_6, B_1, and C—and a variety of psychological problems in children, including learning disabilities, antisocial behaviors, and other behavioral problems.[3] (Unfortunately, such scientifically sound insights into the mental health of America's youth have gone virtually unheeded by state and federal agencies over the past two decades.)

This research fits in well with my own clinical experiences with autistic children, particularly in terms of the nutritional deficiencies we have identified and how they correspond with behavioral problems in these children. Note that, with the exception of vitamin B_1, all of the micronutrients cited above as important in *Nutrition and Mental Health* may be inadequately supplied by the typical American diet. More important, even when these key vitamins and minerals *are* adequately supplied by diet, the gastrointestinal problems seen in an autistic child tend to impede their absorption and assimilation. Without addressing these problems, an autistic child may consume the best diet in the world without deriving any benefit.

Autism, and perhaps all other neurodevelopmental disorders, is strongly influenced by exposure to environmental toxins and the foods we eat. Although the link between diet and brain function is a subject of intense debate, this much is clear: Diet can directly influence the brain's supply of neurotransmitters, natural chemicals that help transmit nerve messages, reduce stress, and control the brain's "reward" centers.

Much of diet's effect on the mind, moreover, depends on the total environment. While some foods protect against toxic substances (such as lead or PCBs), in a highly polluted environment an unbalanced diet may further impede normal behavior and cognitive functioning. Here the problem is not merely a lack or excess of certain nutrients in the diet, but a dietary imbalance that occurs in the context of environmental pollution.

An added glitch, particularly from a researcher's perspective, is that individuals can vary greatly in their behavioral and cognitive responses to food. Some children who have suffered from early malnutrition later grow to function much better mentally—they register higher IQs and their behavioral problems are fewer than other children with similar early nutritional deficits. The disparity is thought to stem from a variety of causes, including genetic differences and early environmental influences. The basic point here is that we must guard against attempts to draw simplistic connections between nutrition and mental health, for it is anything *but* simplistic.

As we have seen, in early life, a child's exposure to the environment is just as important as diet. The infant's brain undergoes rapid integration in the first few years of life. Drugs consumed during pregnancy, a traumatic birth experience, and lack of breastfeeding in early life have all been shown to significantly impair brain development in early life, all three associated with an average drop in IQ of 10 points or more. As I mentioned previously, one out of every ten newborns here in the United States has been exposed to toxic narcotics in the womb.

It is difficult to reverse the effects of early environmental insults to the brain. And if a child is born into the world with some degree of abnormal function, a diet and lifestyle that fail to promote brain health will only exacerbate the handicap. The good news is that for autistic children, food can be a vehicle for healing. Of course, parents must also remember to "feed" their child with a diverse range of brain-stimulating experiences—reading, singing, playing music, building complex structures, running, romping, wrestling, and stimulating the child's brain in numerous ways. Focus on feeding the *whole person*.

Figure 8-1

Is Your Child's Brain Malnourished?

Many authorities have dismissed claims that vitamin and mineral deficiencies are undermining the cognitive potential of American children. Clinically obvious deficiencies of these micronutrients, they point out, are unusual in the West. On the other hand, marginal or *subclinical* deficiencies may be widespread. For instance, one study in a New York hospital found that over two thirds of 200 randomly selected children had one or more deficiencies in essential vitamins and minerals.[4]

In 1988, the British medical journal *Lancet* reported on a survey of ninety school children ages twelve and thirteen. The children were found to be eating far less than the recommended dietary allowance (RDA) of certain micronutrients. Over the course of eight months, the children were given a multivitamin-mineral supplement, placebo, or no supplement. By the end of the school year, while nonsupplemented and placebo children showed no change, the children receiving the supplement significantly improved their scores on tests of nonverbal intelligence.[5]

Using Supplements for Nutritional Healing

Our treatment program is highly individualized, tailored to the needs of each child. Beyond a child's diet, a number of nutritional supplements can be used to address specific nutritional deficiencies, as well as allergies, digestive and immune dysfunction, and other problems.

First, malabsorption needs to be treated vigilantly. We give our autistic patients both nutrients and "nutriceuticals" to help rejuvenate their digestive tracts. The products used to heal the dysfunctional gastrointestinal tract include digestive enzymes, glutamine, zinc, aloe vera, bioflavonoids, and probiotics, which work together to encourage the growth of small intestinal cells (enterocytes) and help to heal the walls of the gut.

We also select from a comprehensive, broad array of supplements, including multivitamins, certain B vitamins, and a special mineral preparation; essential fatty acids including gamma-linoleic acid, alpha-linoleic acid, and DHA (Neuromins®); and a derivative of 10-decanoic acid, helpful for treating seizures and for maintaining the integrity of neuronal cell membranes.

Other supplements include NADH (a coenzyme found in all living cells), coenzyme Q10 (ubiquinone), melatonin (a highly effective "scavenger" of free radicals in brain tissue), lactoferrin, glutathione, N-acetyl cysteine (NAC), L-glutamine, acetyl-L-carnitine, S-adenosylmethionine (SAMe), alkylglycerols (derived from shark liver oil), and various precursors to deficient neurotransmitters. We administer powerful antioxidants that help diminish the action of free radicals, including DMAE, MSM, and an Ayurvedic herbal combination known as Amrit Kalish, as well as the classical antioxidant supplements such as glutathione and vitamins C and E.

Several other "alternative" therapies such as gotu kola and gingko biloba have been shown to be useful in supporting brain function. Ginkgo biloba has been studied extensively, mainly in adults. Our clinical observations suggest that this herb is entirely safe for children, and that it likely plays a favorable role in the recovery of normal brain function for these children.

Radical Protection Against Toxins

All drugs, chemicals, pesticides, herbicides, and pollutants (xenobiotic compounds) must be detoxified or biotransformed in order to be excreted from the body. The biotransformation and detoxication of these chemical compounds take place in the liver. This occurs in two major phases. During phase I, or *functionalization,* foreign compounds are hydrolyzed into water-soluble compounds. Part of this process involves conversion to more or less potent compounds than the parent compounds to render them ready for the next stage of processing. During phase II, or *conjugation,* metabolites produced in phase I are combined with endogenous molecules and become less toxic, thus more readily excreted.

A variety of nutrients and phytochemicals (natural plant-derived compounds or substances) plays a significant role in both phases of the metabolism of drugs and foreign compounds. Most of these stimulate both phases of detoxication. Some, however, stimulate one phase far more than the other, and this fact can be exploited to therapeutic advantage. Nutrients may also stimulate the breakdown and excretion of xenobiotic compounds, and help reduce absorption of these toxic chemicals through the digestive tract.

Antioxidants provide the body's best line of defense against xenobiotics, many of which form harmful free radicals in the body. Thus antioxidants can reduce damage caused by these environmental pollutants. The antioxidant enzymes (superoxide dismutase, catalase, and glutathione peroxidase) are the body's first line of antioxidant defense. The body's second line of defense against free radicals consists of nutrient-derived antioxidants such as vitamins C and E, beta-carotene, some amino acids, glutathione, the DNA bases, and the circulating metalloproteins ceruloplasmin and transferrin. If any of these antioxidant substances are deficient, incomplete metabolism of xenobiotics will result, leading to prolonged chemical action or side effects from incomplete chemical metabolism.

The relationships between such nutrients and the metabolism of xenobiotics are complex. Let's take a quick look at the major antioxidants and their functional roles in the detoxication process.

- **Vitamin C** (ascorbic acid, ascorbate) is a highly versatile antioxidant, as well as an antitoxin. The human species apparently lost the ability to synthesize this nutrient from glucose early in primate evolution, some 60 million years ago. Thus, in humans, the entire complement of vitamin C must be obtained from the diet, and it appears that considerable quantities may be required for optimal antioxidant protection. The presence of foreign compounds increases vitamin C excretion through the urine. High doses of vitamin C have generally been considered nontoxic except for gastrointestinal symptoms experienced by some subjects. At least one study has also shown that vitamin C also improves autistic behavior in some children; this is likely due to the free-radical scavenging effects of the vitamin, which would reduce oxidative stress in these individuals.[6]

- **Vitamin E** (tocopherol), a fat-soluble vitamin, rivals vitamin C as a fighter of free radicals. Vitamin E helps protect lipids (fats) and other vulnerable membrane constituents from oxidative damage. One molecule of vitamin E can effectively protect up to 1,000 membrane lipid molecules from peroxidative attack. Vitamin E cannot be synthesized in the body and should be supplied in the diet in proportion to the fatty acid content of the diet. Low dietary vitamin E intake has been specifically linked with a variety of free radical–mediated degenerative pathologies, all characterized by increased membrane lipid peroxidation. Animal studies have also shown that vitamin E markedly enhances endurance during heavy exercise. Reports of adverse symptoms from large doses of vitamin E abound in the literature, but are largely subjective and based on limited observations.

• **Selenium** works synergistically with vitamin E, which is why you find supplements that often contain both micronutrients. Selenium is essential for the activity of glutathione peroxidase, an integral part of the body's antioxidant enzyme system. As such, selenium protects cells from peroxide-producing reactions—the excessive production of hydrogen peroxide, for example, which can be very destructive. Selenium is also an immune stimulant and may counteract the toxic effects of cadmium, mercury, and possibly other heavy metals. Selenium itself, however, is toxic at high doses, so more is not necessarily better.

• **Beta-carotene** (pro-vitamin A) is a lipid-soluble antioxidant which aids in the control of free radicals by quenching single oxygen molecules and preventing them from forming additional free radicals. It has also been shown to be helpful in preventing the formation of nitrosamines in the stomach and other free radicals elsewhere in the body. Beta-carotene as a supplement may work best in the presence of other carotenoids, which can be provided by a fruit- and vegetable-rich diet.

• **Zinc,** a potent trace element, plays an important role in the functioning of the antioxidant enzyme superoxide dismutase. Zinc stabilizes biological membranes and provides protection against peroxidative damages. Zinc is particularly important for autistic children, since it has powerful effects on the hippocampus, an area of the brain involved in the processing of memory, cognition, and emotion. Like selenium, though, one must guard against taking too much zinc, since the element easily becomes toxic at higher doses.

• **Glutathione** is an antioxidant "tripeptide" composed of three amino acids: glycine, cysteine, and glutamic acid. It is the most abundant antioxidant found within your body cells, and its relative supply within cells is heavily influenced by other antioxidants such as vitamins C and E, and by the body's overall toxic burden. Glutathione can readily bind or *conjugate* with a variety of metabolites, thereby serving to increase their water solubility for subsequent excretion in the urine. Glutathione is an extremely versatile antitoxin, particularly in the lungs and liver, where most detoxifying reactions occur. You can also boost your glutathione levels indirectly by taking substances such as N-acetylcysteine and whey proteins.

• **B vitamins** are typically associated with energy, but their roles also include detoxication and healthy functioning of the immune and nervous systems. These vitamins include thiamin (B_1), riboflavin (B_2), niacin (B_3), pantothenic acid (B_5), pyridoxine (B_6), and cobalamin (B_{12}). Niacin, as a vasodilator, has an effect on lowering lipid levels and possibly on releasing toxins from body tissues. With increased doses of niacin, there is a progressive elimination of pollutants stored in the fat. As cofactors (nutrients that work in tandem with other nutrients or enzymes), several of the B vitamins play critical roles in supporting liver detoxication. Other vitamins and minerals may be indicated on an individual basis to aid the antioxidant support enzymes or to bolster immune function.

Nutritional Supplements for Autistic Children

Many nutrients serve both as antioxidants to aid detoxication, and as essential building blocks for the brain and nervous system. While I use the nutrients above to support the body's detoxication process, I also prescribe a broader regimen of nutritional supplements for autistic children. This regimen is different for each child, depending on individual needs. What follows is a general list of the supplements I most frequently recommend for autistic children.

One caveat before listing these nutrients. Although some forms of these nutrients are available in health food stores, I do not recommend putting together a supplementation program on your own, without medical supervision. I have not provided dosages here, because these also vary from one patient to another. Moreover, higher than normal doses of these nutrients may be required to have the desired therapeutic effects. We perform a number of laboratory tests to uncover the imbalances in each patient. This regimen must be carefully fine-tuned according to the needs of each child, throughout the course of his or her treatment.

• **Multivitamin and mineral preparation**. This is an age-specific combination of essential vitamins and minerals, adjusted according to each patient's needs.

• **Antioxidants**. Antioxidants work to neutralize free radicals, charged particles that can damage the tissues of the brain and nervous system. Autistic children tend to have higher than normal levels of free radicals, which can damage the tissues not only of the brain and nervous system, but of every organ system in the body. Important antioxidants we include are vitamins C and E, beta-carotene, and glutathione. Pycnogenol® (pine bark extract) is another excellent antioxidant which crosses into the brain. It contains oligomeric proanthocyanidins (OPCs), flavoids that serve as highly potent antioxidants.

• **Vitamin B$_6$ (pyridoxal-5-phosphate).** This vitamin has many important effects in the body, especially in DNA synthesis, fat and protein metabolism, neurotransmitter function, and nerve cell metabolism. Vitamin B$_6$ supplementation is especially important for autistic children, since autism has been associated with a vitamin B$_6$ deficiency in some studies. In one study by Rimland, behavioral symptoms in a group of children with autism improved when they received vitamin B$_6$, and worsened again when the treatment was stopped.[7] A later follow-up study confirmed the correlation between vitamin B$_6$ supplementation and improvement of autistic behavior in this group of children.[8] Vitamin B$_6$ in therapeutic doses can cause side effects such as sound sensitivity, enuresis, and irritability, which may be improved by administering magnesium at the same time.[9]

• **Dimethylglycine (DMG).** This is a naturally occurring molecule found in human cellular metabolism. It is used to make sarcosine, which is needed to make the neurotransmitter acetylcholine. DMG is an important element in DNA synthesis, as are the amino acid methionine, choline, and several neurotransmitters and hormones. Research suggests that DMG supplementation may also help control epileptic seizures.[10] In anecdotal reports, DMG has been shown to benefit autistic individuals.

• **Phosphatidylcholine**. This is a phospholipid that yields choline, which is needed for the production of the neurotransmitter acetylcholine, essential for proper brain function. Phosphatidylcholine also happens to be highly beneficial for liver function, which is so important in treating autism. In Germany, it is used to treat a wide range of liver disorders.[11] Though it is found in certain foods, such as legumes, grains, egg yolks, liver, soy, and some vegetables, the typical "autistic picky eater" likely does not get enough of this compound through his diet.

• **Essential fatty acids.** These nutrients play fundamental roles in the immune, endocrine, circulatory, and nervous systems. As structural components of membranes, essential fatty acids help form a barrier that keeps foreign molecules, viruses, yeast, fungi, and bacteria outside of cells, and keeps the cells' proteins, enzymes, genetic material, and organelles (small organs) inside. They also help regulate the traffic of substances in and out of our cells via protein channels, pumps, and other mechanisms. They also help form hemoglobin from simpler substances, keep exocrine and endocrine glands active, make joint lubricants, and are precursors of prostaglandins (short-lived hormone-like substances that regulate blood pressure, platelet stickiness, and kidney function). They help transport cholesterol and generate electric currents that regulate heartbeat. Finally, fatty acids help the immune system fight infections by enhancing peroxide production, and help prevent the development of allergies. Your daily diet is one source of essential fatty acids. In most cases, however, it is impossible to get the optimal amounts of these vital nutrients from your diet, and thus supplementation is required. The major fatty acids are summarized in Figure 8-2.

Figure 8-2

Fatty Acid Supplements You Need to Know About

Gamma-linoleic acid. This is an essential omega-6 fatty acid, necessary for many functions in the body, especially the nervous system. Again, the typical autistic diet is devoid of this fatty acid. Borage oil, black currant extract, and evening primrose oil are excellent sources of this fatty acid.

Alpha-linoleic acid. This omega-3 fatty acid can support brain and immune function. Flax oil is a major source of alpha-linoleic acid. However, many individuals have difficulty utilizing flax oil due to enzyme deficiencies. Alpha-linoleic acid is ideally converted into eicosapentanoic acid (EPA), which then becomes docosahexanoic acid (DHA). For individuals who cannot metabolize alpha-linoleic acid, the use of fish oil (or purified EPA or DHA) may be preferable.

Docosahexanoic acid. This fatty acid, converted from EPA, plays a very important role in the development and function of the nervous system. DHA is needed by the body's most active tissues—the brain, retina, adrenal system, and testes. Some data indicate that mood and cognition are critically dependent on this fatty acid, which is in extremely short supply in the typical American diet. Fish oil is an excellent source of DHA, though one must guard against poor-quality fish oil supplements that are heavily oxidized or loaded with mercury.

- **Calcium EAP (colamin phosphate).** This is a synthetic "chemical" nutrient that was developed in Europe, to aid in healing damaged neurons by healing the cell membrane. Colamin appears to act as a "sealing substance" that heals nerve tissue.

- **Lactoferrin.** This immune-regulating substance is a natural product from cow's milk; a similar compound is found in our saliva and urine. It has been found to help some autistic patients, owing to three different possible mechanisms: It improves the membrane potentials of nerve cells, decreases autoimmune responses, and stimulates nerve growth factors.

- **NADH (Enada).** This is a coenzyme, found in all living cells, that plays a key role in energy production. It has been shown to increase the production of neurotransmitters, and thus may be especially beneficial for autistic patients.

- **Decanoic acid.** This is related to an anticonvulsant drug called valproic acid, a derivative of this type of fatty acid. The fatty acid has been shown to help seizure disorders.

- **Octacosanol (prometol).** This is a long-chain "alcohol" nutrient extracted from wheat germ oil. It has shown benefit in certain neurological conditions such as Parkinson's disease and seizures.

- **Glutathione.** As I noted earlier in this chapter, glutathione is a highly potent antioxidant produced in the liver, where it works to detoxify harmful chemicals so they can be excreted from the body. All children with autistic syndromes should take glutathione, because of its ability to detoxify chemicals and heavy metals in the body. It is also crucial for healthy function of the nervous system. Some children, however, will not tolerate this substance very well.

- **N-acetyl cysteine (NAC).** Supplementation with this important antioxidant and chelator of heavy metals may have beneficial effects on many neurodegenerative diseases. The possible benefits in autism are significant without any side effects. NAC is also a precursor to glutathione (see above), so providing the body with NAC helps elevate glutathione levels in the liver, lungs, kidneys, and bone marrow.

- **Melatonin.** This neurohormone is produced by the pineal gland, a cone-shaped structure in the brain. Melatonin regulates sleep cycles, stimulates the immune system, and also functions as a highly potent antioxidant. There is some early evidence in a few autistic patients that low-dose melatonin can improve behavioral symptoms. Much more research remains to be done in this area, especially in relation to the long-term effects of melatonin supplementation. (It is widely assumed that older individuals benefit more from melatonin supplementation than younger individuals.) Nonetheless, we know that melatonin is a safe therapy if conducted during a relatively brief, trial period.

• **Alpha-lipoic acid.** This highly dynamic nutrient plays a central role in mitochondrial function, and helps to regulate two key enzymes that convert food into energy. It is a superb antioxidant that penetrates into the brain, and works by enhancing the antioxidant abilities of other key antioxidants—vitamin E, vitamin C, and glutathione. Lastly, because alpha lipoic acid binds to heavy metals, it may have a significant beneficial role in autism. There are no side effects in taking this nutrient. Recent studies show it to increase the sprouting of new nerve cells in the nervous system.

• **S-adenosylmethionine (SAMe).** This is a natural metabolite of the amino acid methionine. It has been synthesized and utilized in other countries (mainly Italy, where it was discovered in 1952) to treat various problems involving brain function. It plays a key role in a process called "methylation," in which a single carbon unit (a methyl group) is added to another molecule, a process that is especially important in the synthesis of brain chemicals.[12] SAMe also protects brain cells from damage. It has been shown to help in nerve cell regeneration. It is important because it is essential for the manufacture of glutathione and other sulfur-containing compounds in the body. It may also have a place in the treatment of children with autistic spectrum disorders, since it aids the healing process of the damaged central nervous system.

• **Alkylglycerols.** This chemical compound is natural in shark liver oil, called squalene. Squalene contains nervonic acid, another essential fatty acid that helps to build nerve cells. This is a natural product with no known side effects or toxicities.

• **Gotu kola.** This herbal preparation is a "brain tonic," improving blood flow and function of the brain, and stimulating the central nervous system.

• **Ginkgo biloba.** This nutrient, from the leaves of the ginkgo tree, improves circulation and oxygenation of the brain. Used as an extract, gingko biloba has been shown to improve cognitive functioning, though the clinical research to date has focused on adults or older individuals.

• **Acetyl-L-carnitine (ALC).** This is a molecule made up of acetic acid and L-carnitine bound together, a reaction that naturally occurs in the brain. ALC behaves much like the neurotransmitter acetylcholine, which helps control memory and proper brain function.[13] It also functions in the body to improve mitochondrial function by improving utilization of fats. It has been shown to help various functions in the brain such as the synthesis of nerve growth factor receptors. It also improves energy production in brain cell mitochondria, and protects neurons from injury.

• **DMAE (dimethylaminoethanol).** This nutrient occurs naturally in the body, and acts as an antioxidant in the brain.

• **MSM (methlsufonylmethane).** This is an antioxidant and anti-inflammatory compound that has great therapeutic potential as a treatment for the inflammatory process occurring in the tissues of all autistic patients.

• **Coenzyme Q10.** This compound is essential for cellular energy production throughout the body. It is a powerful antioxidant that behaves in the body much like vitamin E. It helps oxygenate tissues and stimulates the immune system. It has been discussed in autism because of its antioxidant and mitochondrial-stimulating effects.

• **Vitamin B_{12}.** This nutrient improves neurologic function, helps prevent nerve damage, and plays a role in the production of the neurotransmitter acetylcholine, which has to do with learning and memory. Vitamin B_{12} supplementation is especially important in autistic children since a B_{12} deficiency is often caused by malabsorption, which is so widespread among autistic children.

• **Folic acid.** It is essential for the formation of red blood cells, energy production, and immune function. The neurological aspects of this nutrient have led to clinical trials in autistic patients. There have been reports of its great success in certain cases.

• **Trental**. This drug's effect on the cytokines of the immune system is important in the autistic spectrum disorders. It lowers TNF-alpha, IL-1, 6, and 8, and inhibits TH-1 cells; it helps control autoimmune processes, and by inhibiting TH-1, there is a decrease in cytokines produced by TH-1 cells. Side effects may include nausea, bloating, dizziness, headache, drowsiness, and blurred vision.

• **L-glutamine.** This is a form of the amino acid glutamine, which is so important for proper mental function. In the brain it is converted to glutamic acid, and also increases the amount of GABA, both of which are necessary to sustain proper brain function.

• **Vinpocetine.** This product comes from an herb, and has been on the market in Europe for years as a "smart drug." It improves oxygen and blood flow to the brain cells, increases oxygen used by the brain, and raises the local amount of serotonin in the brain.

• **Picamilon.** This is a product from Russia that combines niacin and GABA; its primary effect is to increase blood flow to the brain.

• **Amrit kalish.** An Ayurvedic herbal combination with a fabulous antioxidant potential that is 1,000 times greater than vitamin E or C. It is able to cross into the brain.

• **Curcumin (turmeric).** Turmeric is a bright yellow powder, made from the root of curcumin. This herb has many important functions in autistic patients. It is highly effective as a protector against lipid peroxidation, and also protects renal tubular cells from injury. In addition, it helps stabilize and balance liver detoxication in these children.

• **Naringin.** This is a flavonoid, a plant pigment with therapeutic properties. In this case an extract from grapefruit has proven beneficial in helping to slow the active phase I detoxication process, which the autistic children so often experience. (As an aside, I should point out that the amounts of this substance found in grapefruit juice are far too low to provide any therapeutic benefit, unless one is gulping down gallons of it.[14])

• **Liver growth factors**. These are liquid fractions of peptides from cells of fetal bovine liver tissue. They are bioactive molecules and are used to stimulate healing and improve function of liver cells.

• **Anthocyanidins**. This group of phytochemicals, or plant-derived substances, are wonderful antioxidants that may greatly support the effects of other antioxidants. The two best-studied examples are grape seed extract and pine bark extract.

• **Lutein, lycopene, and the xanthophylls**. These are very potent plant-derived carotenoids, which makes them close cousins to beta-carotene. There is now good evidence that they protect specific vital structures within the body. For example, lutein is best known for its ability to protect the eyes against degeneration, while lycopene affords protection to the prostate gland, a collecting ground for environmental toxins.

Depending on individual laboratory results, specific supplements may be either added to or substracted from a child's nutritional regimen. This is where professional expertise and a solid grasp of nutritional biochemistry are certainly needed. Be sure that someone on your child's medical team has such a grasp. If your doctor is not supportive, I would urge against self-prescribing based on guesswork or Internet-based education. I have seen far too many people attempt to self-prescribe only to later find that their knowledge was incomplete, and that the supplements they chose were either ineffective or in some way inappropriate.

Let me also reiterate that a sound diet can reinforce the effects of the supplementation regimen. The dietary plan for promoting mental health, as I mentioned earlier, is moderately low in fat and animal protein, and high in grains, beans, and vegetables of all kinds. Simply put, parents need to steer their kids away from junk foods laden with chemicals and toward foods that tend to support normal, healthy functioning.

Jenny's Story

As Jenny Gordon's mother tells it, Jenny—the youngest of four children—was a friendly and happy baby. She charmed everyone with her wide gaze, her hazel eyes, and her curly brown hair. Shortly after Jenny was born, her father left for a three-year tour of military duty in England while her mother, Frieda, struggled to take care of four children alone. Frieda, a plump German housewife with blond hair, rosy cheeks, and a quick laugh, had always been easygoing, inclined to run her household with a relaxed attitude and let the children help her with the chores. At the time, in the midst of a somewhat chaotic household, and because of Jenny's sunny personality—her smiles and her affectionate nature—no one suspected any serious problems.

The only strange thing was that at eighteen months old, Jenny still showed no signs of speech. The family pediatrician said she was probably just a little slower to develop than the other children. He assured Frieda that Jenny would catch up eventually. But as time passed, everyone began to realize that the problem was more serious. A slow change became noticeable in the little girl.

As Jenny grew older, she became more and more distant, avoiding the company of other people whenever possible. She still wasn't speaking, and she communicated her desires to her mother through gestures—she would take her mother's hand and lead her to the water faucet, or the refrigerator, or a window, to show her what she wanted. Frieda was dismayed when she began to realize that Jenny had no awareness of her as another person.

At age four, Jenny had a strangely detached manner, so strikingly different from her sunny nature as a baby. She seemed unable to express love, but instead related to her mother and siblings as objects, to be moved around, ignored, or employed as necessary.

Just after her fourth birthday, Jenny's parents took her to a developmental physician, who suggested that she was not autistic but—as the pediatrician had also concluded—that she was merely suffering from developmental delay. At that time Jenny was also diagnosed with mental retardation. Frieda Gordon was not satisfied with being told to watch and wait. She wanted to help her daughter, not sit around waiting to see what would happen

In August 1998, at age five, Jenny was first diagnosed with PDD by a neurologist. The official diagnosis was PDD-NOS. This was a step in the right direction; however, this neurologist had written several books extolling the virtues of Ritalin, so the first thing he did was to put Jenny on this drug.

Despite their suspicions that something was amiss, Jenny's parents were completely surprised by this diagnosis. Frieda told me later that she had always imagined autism to involve arm flapping, tantrums, head banging, and other difficult behavior—and Jenny did not have any of this. She went to a psychologist for a second opinion. The psychologist confirmed the PDD-NOS diagnosis. "There is no hope. Get yourself a life," she told

Jenny's parents. Though Jenny's father, Joe, suspected that the psychologist might be right, Frieda insisted that there must be some way to help their daughter, who seemed to live in a shell of quiet isolation. Frieda and Joe knew only that they wanted to get back their pretty baby girl with the happy disposition. Frieda told Joe she was not ready to give up.

"There has to be a way of treating this," Frieda thought. Jenny's oldest sibling, her brother Peter, had been diagnosed with a seizure disorder two years earlier. They were doing a nutritional protocol for him. And Frieda thought, there must be something like that for what Jenny has.

In October 1998, Frieda brought Jenny, who was then five and a half, to see me at the Edelson Center. Her cousin had found out about our clinic on the Internet, through a list of doctors who specialize in treating autism.

I discussed our treatment program with Frieda, and I had to be honest with her. I knew that she did not have limitless financial resources. The initial tests would be expensive, and the treatment program would be time-consuming and arduous. But, I told her, I felt it was worth it.

"I can help your daughter," I said. These were the words Frieda had been waiting to hear. She said she was ready. The family would find a way to pull together and make it happen.

The following morning, we ran a battery of tests on Jenny. Later that week, the test results came back, pointing to the classic toxic syndrome of autistic illness. Jenny was suffering from abnormal liver detoxication, malabsorption, overgrowth of candida, and a gastrointestinal parasite called *E. nana*. We found elevated levels of lead, mercury, and tin in her body, as well as various chemical toxins. She also suffered from food allergies.

A week later we began her treatment, a course of therapy which would continue for nearly three years, including detoxification, exercise, chelation therapy, a special diet, and a finely tuned regimen of nutritional supplements. The first step was a one-month detoxification program. Jenny celebrated her sixth birthday in the "detox center." She had a birthday party in our clinic with all her siblings and fellow patients.

Jenny put up a lot of resistance to the program at first. One of the hardest parts of the program, Frieda reported, was getting Jenny to swallow the many nutritional supplements she had to take every day. This was a tremendous ordeal, particularly with four other children to care for, but it had to be done, and Frieda persevered. Jenny could swallow the liquid vitamins and minerals with no problem, but her mother had to break open the capsule supplements, blend them together with apple juice, strap Jenny down, and open her mouth to take them. At first Jenny screamed and fought and refused to swallow, but—like most of the children I have treated—after a few days she got used to it and began to cooperate. She also got used to the sauna and treadmill after a few days. The videos and music helped keep her mind occupied, and after about a week, Jenny got used to her new routine.

Frieda told me she was especially glad to be among all the other families going through the program at the same time. It was easier that children did detoxification together, so they could observe each other. She noticed that the sicker the child was, the more cooperative she was. Once Jenny had gotten used to the program, she cooperated. But as she started to get better, she did not want to stay in the sauna for thirty minutes at a time, or do it four times a day. Frieda said that despite the frustrations, she was glad they were there. "You were right, this program is difficult," she told me. "But it is also rewarding. You meet people with common goals. You feel more normal here than anywhere else."

The first signs of improvement were evident before that first month's course of detoxification had ended. Jenny was already more alert. Before beginning the program, she had a small number of words in her vocabulary—but now she began to use words in phrases. One day she said to her mother, as she tried to find her favorite doll in her toy box, "Over here, help me!" Frieda had never heard her use words like that before. With each passing day Jenny seemed more tuned in, responsive, and aware of what was going on around her. She became more cheerful, and began to rapidly learn new words. "She's becoming the life of the party," her mother told me, ebullient. It was all happening faster than anyone had anticipated.

Recently I spoke to Frieda, and she said the biggest change is that Jenny is speaking so much more, and has much better cognition. "Dr. Edelson, considering the fact that when she was four, she had the cognition of a six-month-old baby, she is doing so well." Jenny has now just turned eight, and her cognition, already that of a five- or six-year-old, is improving rapidly.

Jenny is now able to understand directions and take commands, and above all she is aware of the environment around her. She can recite the alphabet and numbers. If you ask her a question, she responds. If she is tired or hungry, she can tell you what she wants.

The family plans to continue with in-home sauna treatments as often as possible, as well as chelation therapy, vitamins, and nutrients. "We're just taking it day by day," Frieda says.

Compared to some of my patients, Jenny's progress has been slow yet steady over the past three years. "The improvement has been slow, but I don't see anything of the good that's been accomplished going away," Frieda reports. "Whatever healing we see has taken place for good."

Frieda has also been home-schooling Jenny since she was first diagnosed with PDD-NOS. They are doing an in-home ABA program. Frieda admits that this, too, has been difficult with such a large family. But they do their best. She hopes to send Jenny to school soon. Jenny can now process information and read flash cards. She is gradually acquiring the skills necessary for school. Her mother feels strongly that even though Jenny is still, at age eight, a little behind her age group, she has the capacity to catch up. "If we do a little private tutoring on the side, she'll be fine," she says confidently, and I have to agree.

As of August 2001, Jenny's condition had improved by an impressive 56% over a period of two years and ten months, especially given the obstacles her mother has faced in continuing her treatment over the past three years.

Frieda admits to me that this has been an expensive process. Would she recommend the program to other parents?

"Absolutely. The money you're going to save in the long run is far greater than the money you're going to spend. If you start something, the whole key is to try to finish it. If I entrust my child to you, Dr. Edelson, with all your enthusiasm to try to get her better, I have to stick it through until I see the job totally done, whatever that takes. Where else are we going to go? God knows why some kids do well, others don't. We are lucky. As a parent you have to be as fervent as possible, so the child can reach her potential. For me, with five kids, the ideal scenario would be having you, Dr. Edelson, as well as a behavioral therapist, a tutor, and a maid! But if we can't do all that, all we can do is do the best we can."

Frieda's only regret is that she didn't begin Jenny's treatment earlier. While they were waiting for her to "catch up" and learn to speak, she says, they were losing valuable time. She wishes they could have begun the program when Jenny was two or three.

Recently Frieda took Jenny and two of her other children to buy shoes. Jenny walked right into the shoe store, sat down, took off her shoe, and got measured. When asked to take a toy ring out of the jar, she took a handful.

Her mother asked her to put them down and take one, and Jenny did as she was asked. When they left, Frieda told her to say goodbye to the shoe salesman, and she waved bye-bye to him and walked out the door. "My two older kids acted worse than Jenny!" Frieda recounted with a laugh. "He was so impressed. The dentist, the hair stylist, the teachers at school— they have all noticed how quickly she is improving. It's so clear that we're on to something. We are just going to keep doing what we're doing."

Chapter 9

◆

Practical Keys to Getting the Toxins Out

At the Edelson Center for Environmental and Preventive Medicine, on any given day, a cohort of several parents are leading their children through a twenty-day program of biodetoxification—sauna therapy four times a day, combined with exercise and massage, chelation therapy, and a regimen of special dietary supplements. You see children sitting patiently in the sauna listening to Rafi songs, children exercising on treadmills side-by-side with their parents, children taking nutritional breaks to replenish essential vitamins and minerals to help their bodies receive maximum benefit from these treatments.

The centerpiece of my treatment program for autistic children is this biodetoxification process, a demanding yet doable course of sauna therapy, exercise, massage, chelation therapy, and nutritional therapy. This regimen is one of the most rewarding aspects of our program: many parents report seeing marked improvement in the behavioral symptoms of their children within days or weeks of beginning the program. At the same time, in many cases the twenty-day regimen must be repeated more than once for such progress to continue.

How does this process of biodetoxification work? Heating toxic chemicals is the only way to mobilize them and drive them out of the body's fatty tissues and into the bloodstream. This process, known as heat depuration, moves toxic chemicals out of the fat, into the bloodstream, and out through urine, stool, and sweat.

Other key elements of the program are chelation therapy to remove heavy metals from the body, herbal and nutritional strategies for enhancing liver function (balancing phase I and phase II detoxication pathways), and removal of obvious toxic material from the home environment to prevent further toxic exposure.

For a child to successfully complete this program, the family must be willing to participate actively in every aspect of treatment. This therapy requires of both parents and children a great deal of hard work, patience, and endurance. Though children may be initially reluctant, we have found that for most the daily regimen of detoxification soon becomes a "game," and within a few days most children usually come to accept and willingly participate in the treatment.

The Detox Drama

The human body has developed, over the course of millennia, an astounding ability to flush out toxic substances. Some of these toxins are produced inside our body from bacteria and fungi, while others are absorbed into the body through the food, air, and water we take in. In modern times, of course, the body's ability to deal with an increasing toxic burden has become a matter of survival.

As we saw in Chapter 4, the past century has witnessed an exponential rise in environmental toxic exposure. Until about 1800, humans were exposed only to biological toxins and "earth-born" toxins such as heavy metals or those produced by the burning of wood and coal. After 1800, we entered into a period in which human beings began to produce toxic chemicals, or xenobiotics, and to use heavy metals increasingly for industrial purposes. Since the beginning of the industrial revolution, we have witnessed a steady increase in the production of toxic chemicals, to the point where 4 billion tons of these chemicals are released onto the surface of our planet each year, and continue to accumulate in our atmosphere year after year.

According to all medical historical accounts, chronic disease was not a major problem in the early 1800s. The major medical problems then were acute infections and accidents. Over the last two centuries there has been an astronomical increase in cancer, heart disease, arthritis, chronic fatigue, childhood developmental problems, and many immune system diseases and neurodegenerative processes such as Alzheimer's disease.

Biodetoxification is a process by which these toxins (heavy metals and chemicals) are removed from the human body. In effect, we stimulate and support the body's own natural ability to excrete toxins. We take your genetic potential, your built-in capacity to tackle toxins, and amplify it many times over.

Heavy metals are removed relatively easily with the use of medications called *chelators* (although heat therapy can also be of some benefit for this). The chelators we use at the Edelson Center include the synthetic chelators EDTA, DMPS, DMSA, and various natural chelators (lipoic acid, glutathione, and N-acetyl cysteine). In chelation therapy, the patient is infused intravenously or is given an oral or suppository medication that enters the body and binds to the metals. This complex then leaves the body through the urine or stool. The length of therapy varies from patient to patient. This procedure is done on a regular basis until all the heavy metals have been removed.

A more complicated type of detoxification is necessary to remove toxic chemicals (xenobiotics) from the body. These chemicals are stored in the fatty tissues of the body, including the brain. Over the last thirty years, physicians practicing environmental medicine have utilized a process called heat depuration to remove these chemicals. This type of biodetoxification uses a sauna to achieve temperatures of 140 to160 degrees Fahrenheit to mobilize the chemicals from the deep "stores" in the tissues. These chemicals then enter the bloodstream or lymphatic system, and are carried to the liver, where they are processed and made water-soluble. They are then carried out of the liver and leave the body via the intestinal tract, the urinary tract, or the skin and saliva.

During biodetoxification, it is essential that we protect the health of the body's key organs of detoxification—the liver, the bowel, and the kidneys. When we "flush" toxins out of the body's tissues, these organs must work harder than usual to ensure that these toxins are eliminated properly. Thus we must nutritionally support the body's natural detoxication system, and make sure it doesn't get overloaded with additional toxins during this process.

Proper nutrition, as I noted in the preceding chapter, is essential to enhance the liver's ability to process and eliminate toxins. Again, a quick review is in order. The liver not only processes nutrients absorbed via the intestines, but breaks down and eliminates toxins circulating in the bloodstream. Once xenobiotic chemicals are mobilized from the fatty tissue through heat therapy and massage, they enter the blood and travel to the liver for processing.

Now, a diet exceeding individual caloric requirements, or one of excessive food intake, impedes the work of the liver. It becomes overburdened with nutrient absorption, and cannot function as effectively as an organ of detoxication. Also, if chemically contaminated food is eaten, the liver is forced to detoxify these chemicals in addition to the others that are already in the body. The liver may become dysfunctional if overburdened with contaminated foods and mobilized chemicals. This jeopardizes the effectiveness of the therapeutic program.

The bowel (colon or large intestine) is another vital organ of detoxication, working in tandem with the liver. The bowel must be kept flushed, its natural flora nourished, and its muscle tone healthy. Toxins must not be allowed to build up in the colon. Therefore, daily attention must be paid to the elimination of bowel contents. If toxins contained in the stool do not continue to move through the bowel, these substances can be reabsorbed and reenter the bloodstream.

Chemicals circulating in the bloodstream will once again enter the liver for processing, or be redeposited in the body tissues. This adds further stress to the liver, which is already burdened with toxin removal. Chemicals that escape liver detoxication can also cross the blood-brain barrier (if it has been injured, or if the patient is less than one year old), or other cell barriers. This can result in chemicals being reabsorbed into the brain or other tissues.

Last but not least, the kidneys also play a key role in eliminating waste during the detoxication process. Products of detoxication must not be allowed to become concentrated in the urine. Therefore, during this process the patient must consume a minimum of two quarts of water daily, to flush the waste products from the body. Without adequate water intake, kidney and bladder irritation and infection may occur, and chemicals not eliminated may be reabsorbed into the bloodstream.

Key Elements of Our Cleansing Program

At our center, patients spend eight hours daily going through this program, which includes exercise, sauna, massage, and nutritional therapy. The number of days required to remove all toxins varies from patient to patient, but a minimum of twenty eight-hour sessions is usually needed. During this process of detoxification the patient at times may feel dizzy, weak, nauseous, and shaky. The process of removing toxins from the storage depots of our body is often an uncomfortable procedure, because chemicals and metals are getting into the bloodstream and producing acute symptoms. There is no shortcut to getting through this detoxification process.

To achieve depuration, we put children in a sauna of 160 degrees, beginning with ten minutes and increasing to thirty minutes four times a day. The saunas are made of cedar and are chemically nontoxic. Children can listen to music in the sauna.

During this process, exercise improves the circulation so that chemicals can be picked up more easily from the fats and moved to the liver. The patient may use a treadmill or bicycle, or simply run in place. We usually ask the patient to do at least ten minutes of aerobic exercise before each sauna treatment.

After the sauna the patient takes a shower, followed by a massage which usually lasts about fifteen minutes. The massage also helps to move the chemicals out of the fatty tissues and into the circulation. In this sense it is much more than just a "feel good" measure for the young patient—though many of these individuals may in time come to see it as a reward.

The next step is a nutritional support break and rest period before continuing with the program. Nutritional studies indicate that adequate vitamin and mineral intake is necessary for successful detoxification (see Chapter 8). This is accomplished by means of a varied diet of moderate to small portions of less chemically contaminated foods, high in fiber, and low in fat, with carbohydrates composing 60 percent portion of the diet, and proteins not to exceed 20 percent. Detoxification requires the use of oils or high-fiber supplements as needed for bowel regularity and water for peristalsis and proper removal of toxins. Food and water need to be as chemical-free as possible in order to avoid the introduction of new toxins. Nutritional supplements are given to meet the individual need for vitamin and mineral intake during the detoxification program.

The heat therapy program can potentially cause a depletion of body fluids, salt, and minerals, so supplementation of vitamins, minerals, and salts is necessary for the maintenance of cellular balance. A weekly laboratory scan reports the health and activity of detoxication organs, and contains information about the body's mineral status.

Throughout the program patients are monitored by our nurses, who take each patient's vital signs three to four times daily. If patients follow our instructions, problems rarely occur. This is not, however, the kind of process you want to undertake at home alone without medical supervision.

We have found that after twenty sessions, blood levels of chemicals can be reduced by approximately 50 to 70 percent. Our patients often report feeling better shortly after beginning the program. At the same time, parents of autistic children often notice marked behavioral improvement within a few days or weeks.

Environmental control is another important aspect of the biodetoxification program. Exercise, heat, and massage assist the body in the elimination of toxins, but a child's environment and diet are equally important for a successful outcome. Environmental choices include a strict avoidance of pesticides, hydrocarbons, formaldehyde, and other toxic volatile compounds and metals. This avoidance may include restricting travel or hotel stays during the program, for example. Such choices continue to be important long after the program is completed. The chemicals removed during the therapy program can be reabsorbed and cause illness to worsen again. The total detoxification program, then, involves not only the detoxification of the body, but also detoxification of a child's environment, resulting in minimal exposure to chemicals in the food, water, and air. This comprehensive approach allows progress to continue, and optimal health to be achieved.

Keeping Your Child Healthy at Home

As I explained in my first book, *Living with Environmental Illness* (Taylor Publishing Co., 1998, coauthored with Jan Statman), the home can have a tremendous impact on health. It used to be that people were primarily worried about older homes, due to the presence of lead paint. But a family that moves into a new home is essentially entering a milieu of toxic chemicals. For children who don't have a fully functioning liver, these chemicals can pose a major health threat. These children are entering a poisonous environment, one that may bring out an autistic predisposition. Unlike adults, a fetus or a newborn infant has no way to remove himself from a toxic environment.

When it comes to the home environment, I advise people to avoid all petroleum-derived heat sources, insecticides, synthetic carpets and mattresses, and formaldehyde-containing substances such as pressboard and plywood. I also advise removing highly odorous materials such as chlorine bleaches and cleansers, ammonia, detergents, disinfectants, solvents, dry-cleaning materials, lighter fluids, paint, varnish, turpentine, and mineral spirits. In addition, avoid room deodorants, scented fabric softeners, scented washing products, perfumes, colognes, scented hair spray, scented soaps, and cosmetics.

Keep in mind, too, that pesticides (which have been linked with autism) are used extensively inside homes, schools, and workplaces. As a result of this widespread use, children can be exposed to a dangerous degree without ever knowing it. Widespread pesticide pollution has also jeopardized the quality of our food, air, and water supply. It is no wonder, then, that with all these repeated exposures, a large portion of the U.S. population is highly sensitive to pesticides, many of which are chemically similar to the nerve gas compounds developed during World War II. The more these substances enter our food supply and accumulate in our fat tissues, the more we will experience their toxic consequences.

Thus, on top of making the home environment a healthy one, a diet centered on organically grown foods is essential for the nursing mother and for the infant, once the feeding of solid food begins. Organically grown foods are not only a way to keep toxic chemicals out of the diet; they also tend to be significantly higher in nutrients compared to conventionally grown foods.

Once an autistic child has gone through our detoxification program, we strongly recommend that you take certain measures to detoxify the home environment, to avoid once again overloading the body with toxins. Here are some concrete steps you can take to minimize your child's day-to-day exposure to environmental toxins, both during and after treatment.

Clean Air. Buy a HEPA filter to purify the air in your home. Use only nontoxic floor and wall coverings; get rid of old and dusty carpets, or new carpets that may contain toxic synthetic chemicals. Avoid pesticides. Use only nontoxic cleaning agents and water-based products. In the next chapter we will talk more about how you can minimize exposure to toxins and allergens in the home by creating a toxin-free "oasis" for your child.

Clean Water. Filter your water with a reverse osmosis carbon filter, or buy bottled spring water (Evian and Mountain Valley are two trustworthy brands). Don't give your child unfiltered tap water to drink.

Clean Food. Avoid giving your child foods with preservatives, dyes, or additives. Note that even though a processed food says "natural" on the label, it may still contain artificial preservatives. Check ingredients on the label to be sure. Buy only organic or "free-range" eggs, poultry, and meat. Don't cook at temperatures greater than 350 degrees Fahrenheit. Drink only natural liquids such as juice and water; avoid sugary soft drinks such as Coke, Pepsi, and Sprite.

Clean Environment. Stay out of toxic places such as paint stores, Home Depot–type stores that sell compounds used for home renovation, Blockbusters, toy stores, and shopping malls. If you go to a movie, call first and make sure no pesticides have been sprayed within the past week. When driving in the car, keep the windows closed and the recirculation system on.

You can purchase safe alternatives to hazardous household products, at stores selling health products.

Charlie's Story

I first met Charlie Underhill and his mother, Kristen, when they visited our clinic in July 1995. Charlie's parents had divorced five years earlier, and Kristen was a busy single mother, working at three jobs and pursuing a Ph.D. in electrical engineering at the same time. A former marathon runner, she was very interested in health and nutrition, and since her son had been diagnosed with autism, she had spent many hours researching nontraditional treatments for the disorder.

Charlie was six years old, a plump little boy with a gentle, melancholy manner. He did not look at me, but glanced anxiously around the room. Charlie was distant and withdrawn, like many autistic children I have met. He could not have appeared more different from his mother, a smart, determined, fast-talking Southern woman, who had frosted blond hair, wore electric blue running shoes, and drove an SUV. Yet immediately I noticed a sweet rapport between mother and son—they seemed to understand each other, and though Charlie was quiet, he did not seem as emotionally remote as many autistic children do.

As soon as Charlie was diagnosed with autism, Kristen began joining support groups so she could meet other parents of autistic children. She said she didn't need the support—she just wanted to learn all she could, and knew that other parents were the best source of information. It was at one of these meetings that she learned about our clinic.

Kristen had also developed a theory that immunizations had triggered her son's autism, and we discussed this on that first occasion. I told Kristen that I did not think immunizations were the sole responsible agent in causing autism. I did not believe that immunizations were the cause of Charlie's autism, despite the temporal connection between the two events.

"I just don't see what else could have triggered this, Dr. Edelson," Kristen said. "He was an early talker. He was fine before the shots."

I explained that early signs of autism were so subtle that they usually went unnoticed before a child was about eighteen months old.

"I think we can find the cause of Charlie's autism," I said. "We will have to do a thorough examination, medical history, and laboratory tests, as we search for clues. Tell me about how he was first diagnosed."

Kristen told me that Charlie had been diagnosed with PDD by a developmental pediatrician when he was three years old. She had noticed that something was not right for a few months before that.

"I knew something was wrong when Charlie was about eighteen months old, because he would have night terrors," Kristen explained. "I know that's not exclusively autistic, though. And then his language acquisition stalled. He kept getting new words, but at the same time, without it being obviously noticeable, he lost old words."

When Charlie was two and a half, Kristen took him to see a pediatrician because of his night terrors, and because she could not see his speech progressing.

"The pediatrician asked me a bunch of questions," Kristen recalled, "and he said—I will never forget this—'I think we can rule out autism.' I had never heard the word before. Instead he suggested that I talk to Charlie more, say things like 'Look, I'm sweeping the floor.' I guess he thought I was talking to him at too high a level or something!"

Over the next few months Kristen took Charlie to see a child psychologist, a geneticist, and a neurologist. The neurologist said he did not have autism, but was just a late talker. The geneticist said he was not sure, but it could be autism. And the child psychologist said he probably had autism.

Around this time, Charlie's speech was erratic. He could say a sentence if he was having a good day and everything came together. But other times he could not speak at all. Sometimes Kristen gave him little tests. "At times, even if he was really hungry, for example, and I gave him a choice between two of his favorite foods, he couldn't say a word," she recalled. "He just gave up and went away. And I knew he was hungry."

"When I took him to the psychologist, I never thought that would be the diagnosis," Kristen said. "I knew Charlie was smart. If he wanted something, he would go figure it out. He would go to great lengths to figure out how to get things without using words. So I knew he was clever—I just thought his language was slow in developing."

Kristen told me she would never forget their conversation. At first the psychologist did not speak directly about autism. But as she spoke, Kristen began to suspect that her son had a learning disability.

"Finally I said, are you telling me that he's going to need special classes?' " Kristen told me. "And then she finally realized that I didn't know what she was getting at. She said, 'I'm not just telling you he's going to need special classes. I'm telling you he's going to need special schools, and if this had been ten years ago, we would recommend institutionalization, and he's got a 70 percent chance of being mentally retarded."

Kristen's first reaction was anger. She thought, "I'm proving her wrong. She doesn't know my kid." This made Kristin put herself in charge of her son's progress. That is how she came to our clinic—she found out about it through her own exhaustive research.

As Kristen continued to relate to me the events surrounding Charlie's early childhood, one detail in particular caught my attention. When Charlie was two years old, Kristen had undertaken a major six-month renovation of their home. It was during this time that Charlie began losing his language skills, and avoiding eye contact. At the time, Kristen said, she attributed these changes to all the chaos and workers coming in and out of their house. Later, she would tell me that she had come to think it was environmentally related.

In my experience this was a familiar scenario: autism arising in children exposed to unusually high loads of toxic environmental substances during a crucial period of neurological development. But we would have to do tests to determine the extent to which such exposure might have played a role in Charlie's illness.

At one point Kristen, counted thirty different kinds of therapy Charlie had undergone. They had tried FGF growth factor, speech therapy, auditory integration training, sensory integration therapy, music therapy, art therapy, and special tutoring, among others. They did not do behavior modification therapy, because Charlie didn't need it. He did not understand misbehaving, Kristen explained. Charlie always did as he was told, never misbehaving—his problem was that he did *everything* he was told, without questioning it or realizing that he had a choice in how to act.

I discussed with Kristen the possibilities for treating Charlie. She already knew a great deal about the link between environmental toxins and autism. She was convinced that this was the best way to help her son. Kristen expressed her astonishment to me that people like the child psychologist who had diagnosed Charlie could continue to name and identify autism as a behavioral phenomenon, without asking *why* these patterns of symptoms are occurring.

"This is the *only* thing that makes sense," she told me emphatically. "Yet people like the child psychologist keep saying that one of the hallmarks of autism is losing previously acquired skills. Is nobody worried about that? Is nobody asking why? That shocks me. You don't have degenerative brain function loss unless there's something going on."

Kristen told me she appreciated the fact that we focused not on the symptoms of autism but its cause. She was relieved, she said, to have found the Edelson Center. She told me she wanted Charlie to begin treatment as soon as possible.

The next day Kristen brought Charlie in again, and we began a series of lab tests, the first step in designing a treatment program for him. I also did a thorough medical examination and took a detailed medical history of both mother and son.

Sure enough, Charlie's test results showed that he was suffering from an overgrowth of harmful organisms, including klebsiella and candida. Tests also showed that he had elevated levels of a number of toxic substances: aluminum, cadmium, lead, toluene, trimethylbenzene, trichlorethane, styrene, xylene, and 3 methylpentane. Like many of my autistic patients, he also suffered from zinc and iron deficiency, as well as myelin basic protein antibodies, abnormal liver detoxication, and food allergies.

The first step in Charlie's treatment would be our twenty-day course of detoxification, which he began the following month. After this initial intensive course of treatment, Charlie's therapy would continue for at least the next two years, and it is to this determination and persistence that I attribute his remarkable success.

Charlie quickly got used to the sauna, treadmill, chelation, and nutrition regimen. Kristen went through every step with him. She bought a sauna for their home, and exercised every day on the treadmill with her son. She went bike riding with him, which he loved. Eventually Charlie came to enjoy the treatments, and even began to seek out the sauna—for him, taking a sauna every day became like taking a bath. He got used to the chelation process, and to taking many pills each day. He also adhered to a special diet to eliminate food allergens, which was the most difficult part for both of them.

Before the twenty-day detoxification program was over, Kristen noticed marked changes in her son's behavior.

Before Charlie began the program, his mother explained, he was unable to reason, and unable to realize that he had a choice in any situation. "He did not realize that you can be mischievous, that you don't have to do something somebody tells you to do, no matter who they are, whether it's a kid or a parent. It didn't matter; he did everything," she said.

Kristen had seen this problem surface also when she offered Charlie a choice between two options. If she said, "Do you want a peanut butter sandwich or a grilled cheese sandwich?" he would say, "a peanut butter sandwich or a grilled cheese sandwich." He did not realize, his mother said, that there *was* a choice.

For the first time, during the course of the twenty-day detoxification program, Charlie was able to make a choice between two things. And he began to think about the world around him in new ways.

"It was the logic piece for him," Kristen told me excitedly. "He began to think about why things happen. During that month we went through detox, I remember one time we were driving through the neighborhood and there was a squirrel going across an overhead wire. Before, Charlie might have looked at it and not said a thing. At the most, he would have said something about the squirrel. He wouldn't even have wondered if that was a strange thing to do or not. But this time it tickled him, seeing that, and he said, 'Why is the squirrel walking on the wire?' Dr. Edelson, that was the first time he had ever asked me a why question. And not only that, he answered it."

Charlie is now twelve and a half. He has been undergoing nutritional therapy, as well as chelation and detoxification as needed, for the past six years. Kristen reports that Charlie's logic and cognition continues to improve. Since we began Charlie's treatment, we have witnessed an amazing 68 percent improvement.

Charlie still acts a bit younger than his age, and he has trouble with social chit-chat; but Kristen is always delighted when people are surprised to find out he is a special needs child. Gradually, he is moving closer to being a normal twelve-year-old.

One of the most amazing changes in Charlie is that he has developed a sense of empathy, which he did not used to have. Kristen recently told me about an incident when Charlie and his six-year-old half-sister Molly were playing on the shore at a lake.

"They have these games that they've made up themselves that they love playing," she said, "and part of it is that Molly will find the biggest rock she can pick up and give it to Charlie and see how far he can throw it. They love this kind of stuff. So she found a really heavy rock that she actually couldn't pick up, but it was close enough. Charlie went and got it, and hoisted it and threw it, and it didn't go very far because it was so heavy. Molly was standing there, curious about how far it was going to go, so that she was actually a little bit in the water. The water ended up splashing her a little bit. She said, 'Charlie, you got me wet!' She kind of lit into him a little bit. And he felt so bad about this, and they were having so much fun playing their little game, that he stepped into the water and splashed water on his own back. 'Oh, look, Molly, I'm wet now too!' he said. It was really sweet. He felt so bad about her being unhappy that he wanted to join her. Yes, that's young behavior for somebody who's twelve. But all the pieces are there. They just need to be developed a little bit more."

Chapter 10

◆

Eliminating Allergens:
An Essential Step

The treatment of autism must extend beyond the clinical setting. Autism must also be managed on a consistent basis by careful elimination of not only the environmental pollutants, but also any *allergens*—the immense variety of substances that can trigger reactions in allergic individuals—from the environment. My program offers specific therapies and guidelines to eliminate both allergens and toxins from your child's environment.

One of the first clues I had that autism might be related to toxic injury was when I made the connection that all autistic children suffer from allergies. This immediately struck me as a critical piece of information. Not only might allergic reactions spark and exacerbate autistic symptoms, I thought, but the fact that so many autistic children also suffer from allergies pointed to a deeper underlying phenomenon—some form of neurotoxic injury.

This approach to treating allergies in autistic children is unusual, because we approach it from two angles. First, we identify allergens and come up with ways for the child to avoid the allergens. At the same time, we work to heal and strengthen the child's immune system, an underlying factor that plays a role in both his allergies and his autism.

When we look at an allergic individual, we are not just looking at one type of abnormal immune reactivity. We study allergy, or sensitivity, by defining it as abnormal reactivity to an environmental characteristic—food, chemicals, bacteria, or inhalants (mold, pollen, dust, and the like). This abnormal reactivity can be an immediate reaction, causing a rash, nasal congestion, stomach pain, watery eyes, wheezing, headaches—or in the case of children with developmental disorders, a whole array of possible behavioral manifestations. Exposure to allergens may also cause a delayed reaction, in the form of joint pains, behavior abnormalities, headaches, muscle pains, depression, insomnia, or other symptoms.

Any organ system can be involved in a "sensitivity reaction." Many individuals who suffer from chronic complaints that are currently being treated with medications to suppress symptoms may actually be suffering from an occult, or hidden, sensitivity reaction.

Traditional allergists do not generally focus on foods or chemicals as a source of allergic reactions. When they do test for food sensitivities, their techniques are not sophisticated enough to pick up subtle sensitivities to foods, and they do not test for sensitivities to chemicals, preservatives, or dyes.

At my Atlanta-based clinic we do two types of allergy testing—skin testing and blood tests that measure the antibodies IgG and IgE. The skin test shows us IgE or immediate-type reactions. The IgG blood test study is somewhat controversial. These are complementary tests, so if any one test shows that you have an allergic reaction to a substance, another test may not; however, the latter result does not contradict the positive result on the first test.

At the Edelson Center we use natural, not pharmaceutical, therapies to treat allergies. We employ a combination of nutritional, detoxification, dietary, and immunotherapeutic interventions. The most effective therapy ever developed is Enzyme Potentiated Desensitization (EPD), which at the present time can only be brought into the United States under the Food and Drug Administration's compassionate use process. This is a vaccine that can, over time, cure allergies. We also use Provocation Neutralization Therapy and a hands-on therapy called the Nambudripad Allergy Elimination Techniques (NAET) to treat allergies, as a complement to EPD therapy.

Above all, we are interested in uncovering the source of a child's autistic symptoms. Any set of chronic symptoms can be based on an immune system reaction and sensitivity. In addition to a thorough physical exam and detailed medical history, we do skin testing and laboratory evaluations to test for allergies. We then design a natural therapeutic program tailored to the biochemical needs of each individual.

This chapter provides an overview of the main therapeutic treatments we use at the center to control—and in some cases even cure—allergies in our autistic patients.

Avoidance of Allergy-Producing Foods

Almost every one of the autistic children I have treated suffers from food sensitivities. Reactions to foods may actually be caused not only by allergies, but by a number of different factors. These include reactions to toxins in food such as spices or curries; reactions to pesticides on fruits and vegetables; allergic reactions to salicylates or chemicals such as caffeine, artificial preservatives, bleaches, or other chemicals; enzyme defects as in lactase deficiency or aldehyde dehydrogenase deficiency; fat intolerance; or irritable bowel syndrome.

The recommended diet to counteract the effects of these sensitivities—as with the regimen of daily nutritional supplements—will vary from one patient to another. We often use a basic dietary regimen called the *avoidance diet* (avoiding foods that trigger reactions); in addition, we occasionally recommend a more involved strategy in which various foods are rotated, known as the *rotary diversified diet*. Both strategies help reduce the chances that the body will react to a potential food allergen. The principal theory behind the use of this diet is that continuous, multiple, and cumulative exposures to commonly eaten foods result in the development of chronic food allergies. Initially the body handles those cumulative and repeated exposures. But over time the body begins to lose its ability to adapt, and food allergy/addiction results. The rotary diet is based on the fact that the gastrointestinal (GI) tract takes three to four days to eliminate a food after its ingestion. If the body is exposed daily to a specific food, this food accumulates in the GI tract—along the twenty-eight feet of the bowel, every few inches there is another exposure of these food substances to digest, utilize, process, and eliminate.

As a result, the body moves into a state of imbalance, a cycle of maladaption and addiction. This maladaption develops not after the first exposure to a food, but only after cumulative and repeated exposures to the offending foods. According to Randolph, maladaption takes on the form of addiction where the body requires the food on a constant basis to maintain feeling well. If the food or meal is missed or delayed, the body experiences withdrawal symptoms, which may be manifested as chronic physical or mental problems. Cumulative previous exposures interact with current food exposures to produce chronic symptoms. These symptoms may fluctuate on and off every day with no obvious relationship to a food or meal.

Rotating all foods, which involves not eating a food more often than once every four days, will spare the body from developing a maladaption or addiction to certain foods. Each spaced ingestion of the food allows the body an opportunity to handle each exposure without developing problems.

On the rotation diet, everything—including foods, beverages, and seasonings—is rotated and not eaten more often than once every four to seven days or longer. A food usually remains in your body three to four days (longer if you are constipated). You are most likely to have symptoms from a food if a second portion is eaten before the first exits the body.

Foods may also be rotated according to their biological food family. For example, if you eat pork on Monday, you cannot eat pork again until Friday. That includes all forms of pork—bacon, roast, ham, and the like. All foods listing "shortening" on the label without specifying vegetable shortening, such as crackers, cookies, and cakes, probably contain pork products, and must be rotated as such.

Here are the basic guidelines for the rotary diversified diet:

- Your child should eat no food more than once every four days.
- Omit all "junk food" from your child's diet, including candies, cakes, cookies, pies, soft drinks, and processed foods containing additives, preservatives, or food coloring.
- Avoid canned foods.
- Use fresh organic or "free-range" foods whenever possible.
- Season only with sea salt (regular salt may contain dextrose and other ingredients).
- Foods may be eaten raw or cooked (steamed, boiled, broiled, baked, or fried). Do not cook at temperatures above 350 degrees Fahrenheit.
- Use spring water in glass containers for drinking and cooking. Bottled spring water is best; reverse osmosis–carbon filtered water is also acceptable. Do not give your child nonfiltered tap water to drink.
- Space meals at least three to four hours apart.
- Your child should not spend longer than one hour at each meal.

Figure 10-1

Recognizing Delayed vs. Immediate Types of Food Allergies

Delayed	Immediate
Multiple foods can be involved.	Rarely more than 1–2 foods involved.
Large amounts of the food are needed to provoke symptoms; reactions may not occur after a single food challenge.	Even trace amounts of food can trigger severe, life-threatening reactions
Reactions occur 2–24 hours after eating reactive foods; rarely, reactions have been reported up to 72 hours later.	Reactions occur 2 hours or less after consumption of offending foods.
Any organ system can be involved in reaction, including the classic allergic areas.	Primarily affects skin, airway, and digestive system. Classic processes: hives, asthma, eczema, vomiting, diarrhea, and anaphylaxis.
Very common in both children and adults; causes, provokes, or worsens over 50 medical problems.	Rare in adults.
Addictive cravings and withdrawal seen in 20–30% of cases.	Addictive cravings never seen.
Because of multiple foods and delayed onset of symptoms, the offending foods are rarely self-diagnosed.	Offending food is often diagnosed because of immediate reaction.
Allergic foods are favorite foods. Symptoms clear after avoidance for six months.	Allergic food is a rarely eaten food. A permanent fixed allergy.
IgE RAST negative; IgG positive (type II) often.	IgE and skin test positive (type I) reaction.
IgG food immune complexes (type III) and cellular (type IV) reactions common.	IgG not involved.
Sensitized lymphocytes, eosinophils, platelets, release of leukotrienes prevalent.	Mast cell release of histamine and tryptase involved.

Mold Allergies

Because we cannot see them, we tend to forget that molds are everywhere. Mold is one of the main triggers of allergic disease. The air is filled with mold spores, and these spores, like pollen, can cause allergic symptoms when they land on your nasal and bronchial mucosal membranes, or on your skin. In fact, they cause more protracted symptoms than pollens, but because their symptoms are often also more subtle, they may be hard to identify as allergies.

Mold allergy may be responsible for "classic" allergic symptoms such as wheezing, nasal congestion, abdominal pain, or headaches; but they may also trigger "nonallergic" symptoms that have failed to respond to any type of therapy whatsoever.

Mold prevalence, however, changes with time, as new molds are always developing. New molds get introduced into the atmosphere probably from a variety of sources, one example being excavation for housing tracts and roads. New molds are introduced into the air that were never present before, and once there, they do not disappear when the excavation site is covered over, but instead they flourish in their new environment and trigger allergic symptoms. Molds have seasonal fluctuations in quantity as well as quality. They peak during pollen season, but turning up the heat and humidifier in winter encourages the growth of mold.

Enzyme Potentiated Desensitization

Enzyme Potentiated Desensitization (EPD) is a technique using extremely small doses of allergens to desensitize the patient against his allergies. The doses used are much smaller than those employed in diagnostic skin testing. An enzyme called beta glucuronidase is used as a *biological response modifier* to increase and alter the effect of these antigen extracts.

This method was first developed in 1966 by U.K. researcher Dr. Len McEwen. He found that a single dose of grass pollen with beta glucuronidase could be as effective as a long course of conventional desensitizing injections. The technique was subsequently adapted as a treatment for other allergies. Since the dose of allergen needed is much smaller than that used for conventional desensitizing injections, this treatment is also much safer. Beta glucuronidase is an enzyme present throughout the human body. For EPD the dose of enzyme used is less than that contained in one cubic centimeter of blood from a healthy person. Beta glucuronidase is released into the tissues during inflammation or allergy in quantities greater than those used for EPD. The treatment exploits a natural phenomenon by using accurate and very low doses.

EPD stimulates the immune system, leading over time to the control of allergies to foods, inhalants, and chemicals in over 80 percent of suitable patients, over a period of several years.

Neutralization: Combining Skin Testing and Antigen Challenge

In this method, each allergen is first tested separately by intradermal injection of changing doses, to find the lowest dose that provokes a skin response. This is called the neutralizing dose. The neutralizing dose is used regularly by injection or under the tongue to give protection from ordinary exposure to the same allergen for sometimes two hours, sometimes up to two days. In the hands of a competent doctor, this method has proved much safer than conventional immunotherapy. Neutralization can work for most allergens, including foods, but the results for wheat and milk are generally poor.

The main advantage of this method is its immediate effect. Short-term (up to three months) trials of neutralization versus "placebo" have demonstrated the efficacy of this treatment, although the true success rate may be rather less than for EPD. Moreover, this therapy does not provide long-range relief. The disadvantage is that neutralization, unlike EPD, does not lead to a cure. The drops or injections may need to be continued indefinitely. Also, the neutralizing points may change so that the previous dose causes symptoms and retesting is necessary, sometimes within three months. This can be tedious and expensive if many allergens are combined in a patient's treatment.

Nambudripad Allergy Elimination Techniques (NAET)

NAET, which was discovered by Dr. Debby S. Nambudripad in the late 1970s, is used throughout the United States and Europe. It is a completely natural, noninvasive holistic treatment that incorporates diverse techniques from various medical disciplines, for the purpose of treating and eliminating all types of allergies. This approach can never lead to long-term control, however, and there is no scientific proof of its efficacy. The theoretical basis of NAET is a combination of hands-on techniques to eliminate energy blockages and to restore the body to a state of balance. This approach combines sophisticated knowledge of the brain, cranial nerves and nervous system, organs, and tissues of the body, with kinesiology, chiropractic techniques, and Chinese medical principles. Kinesiology is a technique of measuring muscle weakness produced by energy obstructed in particular spinal nerve routes by an allergen. Chinese medicine highlights the concept of homeostasis, or maintaining a dynamic, harmonious state of balance among the body's energies and functions.

Ozone Therapy

Another promising technique that we use to treat allergies—as well as other symptoms of autistic spectrum disorders—is ozone therapy. Seven thousand doctors in Germany use ozone to treat a large number of chronic illnesses. Ozone is produced when ultraviolet light from the sun irradiates molecular oxygen. In nature, it forms a protective curtain over the earth during daylight hours. At night there is no protective curtain. Ozone is a blue gas at room temperature, with each molecule composed of three oxygen atoms joined together. In the air or the body, it is quickly converted to oxygen and the superoxide anion.

Ozone works in the body by forming stable molecules called ozonides with molecules of the body. These ozonides can penetrate cell membranes and speed up reactions of all sorts. In autistic children, ozone confers the following purported benefits: increases oxygen in tissues; opens arteries for improved circulation; modulates the immune system; normalizes hormonal and enzyme output; neutralizes chemical toxins by oxidizing them; boosts the production and activity of antioxidant enzyme systems; neutralizes free radicals; and improves brain function. This treatment has almost no side effects.

The process of administering ozone therapy is called autohemotherapy. Some blood is drawn from the patient's vein, and is then mixed under sterile conditions with a very specific amount of ozone gas, calculated based on the individual's specific condition. It is then dripped slowly back into the patient.

Creating an Oasis

One of the most important things you can do for your child is to set up an "oasis" in your home—a room with filtered air, free of environmental toxins. Potential allergens in your home may include molds, mites, dust, pesticides, plastics, paint, and a host of other ubiquitous household substances. An "oasis" gives your child a place to get away from chemical exposures. The time a child spends in the "oasis" is "rest time" the body has away from chemical exposures, thereby allowing the immune system to recover from the sensitivity. Here are some specific guidelines for creating an oasis in your home.

- **Floor.** Ideally the floor should be a wood floor, but not freshly varnished. Remove all rugs and carpets. If the floor is plywood (or vinyl tile), cover with a cloth or Mylar "space blanket," since plywood is glued together with resins made of petrochemicals. Wash floor with Borax or baking soda and water. Cover heating vents with aluminum foil or Mylar, and tape with masking tape. Cover floor with cotton rugs or cotton sheets and towels.

- **Walls.** Do not repaint now. Wash down walls with Borax or baking soda and water. Avoid using a room with vinyl wallpaper or adhesives containing anti-termite insecticides. Bare, unsealed pine surfaces should be covered with a cloth if fumes are too strong and fresh. Remove all clothes from closet in room, especially polyester or dry-cleaned clothes. Your child should be exposed only to cotton sheets, curtains, and clothing.

What to put in your "oasis":

- **The filter.** This is the most important item in the oasis. It should be turned on and left on constantly, and the door closed to the oasis. Use a HEPA air filter.

- **The bed.** The mattress, pillow, and box springs should not contain sponge rubber urethane foam or synthetic fabrics. Some mattress coverings have odors to their print dyes. The best is a 100 percent cotton mattress. The bed frame should be all metal or wood, cleaned with Borax or baking soda. Or the mattress can be placed directly on the floor. Alternatives are enclosing the mattress and box springs with aluminum or Mylar, sealed at seams with masking tape. Blankets, pillows, and sheets should be 100 percent natural cotton (not "drip dry" or "permanent press" treated). Folded cotton towels or feather pillows (if not allergic to feathers) may also be used.

• **Furnishings.** The desk should be of wood, glass, or metal. Avoid plastic. The chair ideally should be made of wood; if not, the vinyl area should be covered with a barrier cloth and sealed. Avoid plastic lampshades that will give off odors; clean lamps with Borax or baking soda. The clock should be hard plastic. TV or radio should be black and white, as color TV may give off odors; remove from oasis before going to bed at night. Cover the plastic mouthpiece of the telephone with aluminum foil, or a cotton sock. Use radiant electric heaters or hot water electric heaters only. Remove all toiletries from the oasis, including cosmetics, perfumes, after shave lotions, and scented powders.

In addition to creating this safe toxin-free haven, it is also important to keep your child out of toxic places outside the home. Some of the places to avoid include paint stores, Home Depot–type stores, malls, Blockbusters, toy stores, and possibly movie theaters (call first to make sure no pesticides were sprayed within the previous week).

Evan's Story

Evan Greeley's parents brought him to our clinic two months before his fourth birthday, in March 2000. A slight boy with dark hair and tortoiseshell glasses, Evan exhibited classic autistic symptoms—flapping his hands, uttering little grunts and shouts, suddenly jumping up from his chair for no apparent reason.

Evan's father was in the Air Force, and the family had been stationed in Japan when Evan, then barely three years old, was diagnosed with autism. At that time his mother, Gloria, was eight months pregnant; Evan's father John flew back to the States with their son for tests. They knew something was amiss already, so the actual diagnosis wasn't a complete shock.

"What made you realize there was something wrong, that you had to get your son tested?" I asked.

"He wasn't talking," John explained. "He was almost three. He was always alone, and he seemed to prefer it that way. It was like we were losing him." John was six foot three, a pilot, with a kind face and a crew cut. I could see in his face that this experience with his son had shaken his world.

"And his eye contact stopped. He never looked us in the eye anymore," Gloria added. She was tall and elegant, with no makeup and long dark hair pulled back in a ponytail. She held the baby on her lap, and kept one eye on Evan as she spoke, gently putting a hand on his shoulder whenever he got too restless.

It had been particularly hard on the family because Evan had appeared to be completely normal until he was about two and a half years old.

Gloria explained, "Evan was going downhill, and it was kind of hard to see. That made it more difficult. At first you think you're getting a normal child. Then one day your child is not normal and no one really understands the disability. If my child had been born with Down syndrome or some other disability that is there from the beginning, then we would have known what we were getting. Then you've got your plan. This has been more devastating with Evan because we were suddenly hit with this news that he was autistic."

Evan was diagnosed with autism in April 1999 by a developmental pediatrician, a psychologist, and a neurologist. For a year after the diagnosis, the family—still living in Japan—had tried several therapies with their son, including behavioral modification therapy and sensory integration therapy. But none of them seemed to be very effective. Their son was getting worse, not better. Then, a couple of months before we met, they had spoken to a friend whose fourteen-year-old autistic son had been treated at the Edelson Center several years earlier.

I explained to the Greeleys that I thought I could help Evan. First we would have to do a series of laboratory tests, to evaluate the levels of xenobiotic chemicals and heavy metals in his body, as well as test his digestion, immune system, and liver detoxication system. I would take a detailed medical history from each of them, and perform a thorough medical examination on Evan. Treatment would be an arduous and time-consuming process. The Greeleys said they understood—they were already familiar with my approach, they said, and that was what had brought them here. They said that even though they knew that both tests and treatment would be expensive, they both felt sure this was the right course of therapy for Evan.

The Greeleys had also agreed to spend several months at our clinic in Atlanta if necessary. They were ready to work hard. I explained my theory about how autism is a disease that begins with toxic exposure, that autistic symptoms are produced by a combination of toxic injury and a genetic predisposition to abnormal liver detoxication. We would have to wait and see what the tests showed, but if Evan fit this profile, we would almost certainly be able to help him. Especially because Evan was still relatively young, I told them, I had high hopes for the outcome of his treatment.

As they were getting up to go, John turned to me. "You are the first doctor who has said anything that made any sense," he said, "and who isn't just treating the symptoms. This is the first time we've seen someone who is going straight to the cause of the problem."

When the lab tests came back a few weeks later, they showed that Evan had multiple food allergies, as well as elevated levels of several heavy metals (lead, tin, mercury) and xenobiotic chemicals (xylene, hexane, styrene, pentane). He was suffering from a deficiency in zinc and magnesium, as do many of the autistic children I have treated.

I met briefly with the Greeleys again the next day, and we agreed to go ahead with the treatment, which would begin with our intensive twenty-day course of detoxification therapy. In May 2000, Evan started the program.

Evan did not adapt easily to the detoxification regimen. First, his parents had trouble getting him to take the twenty to thirty daily nutritional supplements that were part of the protocol. Evan screamed and fought, spitting out the juice with which his mother had mixed the contents of the capsules. Gloria changed his diet, but he often refused the new foods. He had always been resistant to new foods, and now he was being given new foods every day. His mother had panic attacks, worrying that he would not be able to eat anything. The family also found it difficult to make the necessary changes in their environment and lifestyle. Like most families, they were not used to having to think about potential toxins and allergens everywhere they went, from the movie theater to the department store.

Though Evan did not like the sauna at first, he soon got used to it and came to accept it. His mother also found it hard to get him to drink enough water while he was in the sauna, and she was always trying new kinds of cups and straws to get him to drink more. It was even more difficult for Evan to adapt to the treadmill. He often wanted to stop before he had been on it for the requisite thirty minutes. His parents had to bribe him, bringing bubbles, treats, and videos to entertain him and coax him through the process. Over time, however, he got used to the regimen and became more cooperative about everything.

Shortly after Evan completed the twenty-day detoxification program, however, his parents noticed two major changes in their son's behavior. The first was that he became completely toilet trained. He had been working on this for over six months, without success. Within a few days of his finishing the detoxification regimen, it happened completely.

The other thing was that Evan had always had a sensitive head. His mother could not shampoo, comb, or cut his hair without his screaming and panicking—"it was like he was being murdered," Gloria said with dismay. They had never been able to take him to a barber, but always had to cut his hair at home. This sensitivity about his head also disappeared soon after the detoxification regimen ended.

"That was amazing," Gloria recalled. "I remember the first time my husband took him to the barber. They came home and I said, 'How was it?' My husband said, 'He was fine.' I almost cried, I was so happy. I put my scissors away, and now he just goes to the barber with everyone else."

The Greeleys also saw smaller changes in their son—Evan's speech began to develop faster than it had before, and he was less foggy and confused, less hasty in his actions.

Since Evan began detoxification therapy, it has been over fifteen months, and Evan has been slowly but steadily improving. Over this period, his behavioral symptoms have improved 52 percent. His teachers always comment on how well he is doing. The changes they have noticed are not sudden and transient, but gradual and pervasive. His teachers are happy with his progress. His behavior is less rigid and stubborn, and his tantrums are less frequent.

The Greeleys moved back to the United States shortly after Evan was diagnosed, to be closer to their families in Virginia and Maryland. They bought a sauna for their home, and now Evan takes a sauna every day. He is still taking many nutritional supplements, which he has grown accustomed to. He still undergoes chelation therapy periodically. His diet has changed permanently; he will never go back to eating the way he did before, Gloria says emphatically. She says the whole family's eating habits are healthier now as a result. He is also undergoing occupational therapy and applied behavioral therapy, and has had auditory integration training. At the same time, the family avoids stores like Home Depot, canceled the exterminator's visit, and generally remains vigilant about protecting their son from exposure to environmental toxins.

"Dr. Edelson," John told me recently, "you were the first person that gave us any hope for Evan, the first one who said, 'I know what causes autism and I can certainly improve it.' That was music to our ears. We appreciated that."

"There is so much to learn with autism," Gloria added. "It can be overwhelming. Every time we turn around there's some other thing to do. You just have to take it one little step at a time. You have to get empowered and you have to figure it out yourself as you go along."

A year and a half into the treatment program, Evan continues to progress, and his parents continue to dream of the day when he will be considered normal and the diagnosis of autism no longer applies.

Afterword

◆

The Health and Healing of Future Generations

We have seen that autism is caused by genetic and environmental factors, a combination of abnormal liver function and neurotoxic injury. The exciting body of research I've presented in this book should incite a renewed sense of urgency. Ecological and mental health are inextricably linked. Why, then, have scientists been so slow to recognize the links between autistic disorders and environmental factors?

One reason is that so little is known about the toxicity of many chemicals present in our environment. We have yet to fully grasp how even very common chemicals—many of which are interacting with other pollutants as well as nutritional factors—are influencing our children's physical and mental health on a daily basis. We have yet to fully understand the magnitude of toxic hazard these substances pose to the well-being of our younger generations, much less to that of generations to come.

Speaking at the 2001 annual meeting of the Learning Disabilities Association of America, National Institute of Environmental Health Sciences (NIEHS) director Kenneth Olden borrowed a metaphor from Judith Stern of the University of California at Davis: "Genetics loads the gun, but environment pulls the trigger." Olden went on to say that "current gaps in our knowledge keep us from preventing the loaded gun from going off again and again."[1] These statements eloquently illustrate the current scientific thinking that genes and environmental pollutants interact within each individual to produce autism and other neurodevelopmental disorders.

Approximately one in every six U.S. children has a neurodevelopmental, learning, or behavioral disorder. I first read that figure in the June 2001 issue of *Environmental Health Perspectives*. The estimate actually comes from a U.S. Census Bureau report published in the medical journal *Pediatrics* in 1993. When this book has been published, nearly a decade will have passed from the time these estimates were published. We humans are often slow to respond to a crisis until it hits us smack in the face—which usually means until it hits home.

This prompts the question: Can we truly afford to wait for costly large-scale clinical studies to provide the definitive answers, the scientific certainty we would all like to have? In light of *what we don't know*, I feel strongly that it would be best to act on an aggressive precautionary basis at this point. Let us assume that, while all the facts have yet to be elucidated, we already know the truth. Environmental pollution is stealing away the minds of our children. The time to act is now, wielding the ultimate form of medicine—prevention. We need to begin taking steps to prevent that "loaded gun" from going off repeatedly. Reducing the ever-growing toxic burden of environmental pollution on our children's health will require major collaborative efforts from numerous agencies and organizations, including the NIEHS, CDC, EPA, and others. Action at the grassroots level will also be needed. We owe it to our children. We owe it to all future generations.

The clinical findings I've presented in this book clearly point to the need for widespread testing of the effects of chemical pollutants on brain development. A similar argument has been presented in "Polluting Our Future: Chemical Pollution in the U.S. That Affects Child Development and Learning," a report published jointly by the National Environmental Trust, Learning Disabilities Association of America, and Physicians for Social Responsibility. The report proposes that government agencies provide testing of the effects of pesticides, food additives, metals, drugs, and other chemicals on the developing brain. This is nothing short of a scientific call to arms, issued by some of the best minds in the country. Until we take this type of large-scale action, we continue to live in what Kenneth Olden calls "a state of toxic ignorance."

A Basis for Optimism?

As evidence for the neurotoxic effects of environmental chemicals on children continues to mount, there has been a surge of interest in environmental medicine. Much of this interest has been sparked by some major environmental episodes in recent decades, such as the health problems experienced by soldiers exposed to Agent Orange in Southeast Asia and the toxic agents used in the Gulf War. The interest has been sparked by tales of entire towns becoming seriously ill—witness the stories of Love Canal and Linley, California, the town near the Pacific Gas & Electric plant whose story was the focus of the recent hit film *Erin Brockovich*. Such dramatic events have helped foster a growing awareness of the dangers chemicals pose to the developing brain, to normal human behavior and basic intelligence.

When you consider the endless stream of mind-poisoning pollutants now entering our environment, it's hard to avoid feeling a modicum of cynicism, particularly with new evidence indicating that these pollutants may be spawning an ever-rising tide of autism and other neurodevelopmental disorders. Nonetheless, there are reasons for hope. The past decade has seen an explosion of popular and scientific interest in the subject of environmental pollution and its impact on children's health. In June 1998, *Environmental Health Perspectives* devoted an entire issue to studies of children and their environment, including several concerned with "neurobehavioral toxicants" such as lead and PCBs (which can damage the developing nervous system of a baby from the earliest stages of pregnancy on).

In the same month, the *Canadian Journal of Public Health* published the proceedings from "What on Earth?: A National Symposium on Environmental Contaminants and the Implications for Child Health," and called for similar action to find ways to prevent toxic substances from harming the brains and nervous systems of children of all ages. Two years earlier, the U.S. Environmental Protection Agency (EPA) had issued a report titled *Environmental Health Threats to Children*. In this report, EPA scientists argued that older standards of safety must be revised or expanded to help protect children living on our increasingly toxic planet. Since the release of that report, the impact of the environment on children's health has become the subject of three bills presented to the House: the Children's Environmental Protection and Right to Know Act, the Children's Environmental Protection Act, and the Pediatric Research Initiative Act.

More recently, the EPA established an Office of Children's Health Protection in response to a series of well-designed studies that documented the effects of chronic, low-level exposure to dietary pesticides and other toxic substances. These substances have been implicated in the dramatic increase of childhood leukemia, brain tumors, and birth defects in the United States over the past twenty years. One can only hope that our government's interest in this all-important area will continue to grow in the coming years.

As a physician who constantly strives to keep abreast of new research, I highly recommend that scientists and laypeople refer to *Environmental Health Perspectives*, a peer-reviewed publication of the National Institute of Environmental Health Sciences, based in Research Triangle Park, North Carolina. In the past year, every issue of this journal has contained a special section on children's environmental health concerns. Also, as of this writing (spring 2002), a new quarterly peer-reviewed journal dedicated solely to children's health issues, the *Journal of Children's Health,* has been announced. It is devoted to reporting on studies of "the unique risks to children from chemical, microbial, radiological, physical and social hazards in their environment." The articles in this new journal will center around whether current exposures to agents in food, air, water, soil, and other media are harmful to or protective of our children's health. These and other research-oriented publications will help foster an improved understanding of environmental health issues among the scientific and regulatory communities.

Concerns about the impact of environmental poisons on children have carried over into the public realm as well, thanks largely to the social consciousness of American celebrities. Actor Robert Redford and vocalist Olivia Newton-John participated in a symposium held in Sundance, Utah, in April 1997, called "Bridging the Gap Between Children's Health and the Environment." That same month, President Bill Clinton issued an executive order demanding increased attention to the protection of children from environmental hazards. The burgeoning movement has also garnered the highly vocal support of actress Meryl Streep, whose own concern as a mother of four led her to raise national awareness toward the adverse effects of pesticides in children's diets.

These and many other developments offer compelling evidence that understanding and protecting our children's physical and mental health from the harmful effects of environmental toxins has emerged as one of the pressing issues on the national agenda.

Effective Therapy by Attacking the Root of Autism

My research at the Edelson Center for Environmental and Preventive Medicine has led me to a bold yet accurate conclusion: Our program for treating autistic children works. My clinical studies have confirmed that this integrated program of detoxification, chelation, and nutritional therapy can be phenomenally effective. When we remove the toxic burden from the body's tissues, and support the liver through nutritional therapy, a child's autistic behavior naturally improves. Over the past several years I have seen many patients improve so dramatically that they were no longer labeled autistic. Many have gone on to successfully attend mainstream schools and live normal, happy lives.

This approach achieves remarkable results because it focuses on the root cause of autism, rather than merely the control of its symptoms. As we have seen, autism is a neurobiological disorder, an illness that involves multiple organ systems. This disorder is triggered by toxic injury during a crucial window of neurological development. In our three clinical studies (which I described in chapter 1), all of our autistic patients suffered from abnormal liver detoxication; allergies to foods, chemicals, or inhalants; and elevated levels of heavy metals and xenobiotic chemicals in their bodies. Most suffered from severe nutritional deficits as well.

All this means that we cannot go back to treating autism by simply trying to correct autistic behavior. We know now that the root cause of autistic behavior is a vicious cycle of neurotoxic injury. Given this situation, we have no choice but to treat autism from the inside outward, working to detoxify the body and strengthen its natural defenses. When this process is carried out with care and expertise, other approaches traditionally used to manage autism become far more effective, and colossal improvements in behavior soon follow.

Until now the major treatments for autism have been mainly palliative, including occupational or behavioral therapy, sensory integration therapy, and even drugs to help keep children's behavior under control. As a result, a child may learn to behave appropriately, but this "learned" normalcy in many cases remains mechanical, not organic to the individual. With this kind of treatment, the child's inner experience does not change much, if at all. A child might still feel as isolated as before treatment, but he has now learned how to appear normal, to behave in a way others behave, even though he may not *understand* why others act as they do.

Although autistic children become more manageable through behavioral modification therapy, they never attain the level of freedom that is born of being able to use one's own mind freely. Over and over again, I've observed that a child who has been liberated from his toxic burden has such a liberated mind. The ABA- or Lovaas-trained child, on the other hand, knows the right things to say to please others—mainly his parents. He may be functioning at a less chaotic level than before, but his mind is still trapped, at least to some degree, in the dark tunnel of autism.

This is not an indictment of Lovaas and other established behavioral modification approaches, all of which have definite benefits. Indeed, I would never recommend going without them. At the very least, these approaches do help stabilize the autistic child. Nonetheless, behavioral modification strategies reap far greater dividends for the autistic child when they're combined with treatments aimed at alleviating the toxic burden in the child's body. To be truly effective, the autistic brain must be liberated from the stranglehold of toxicity that is the hallmark of this disorder.

Healing Sometimes Entails Profound Commitment

A long-term commitment to therapy is vital to the ultimate well-being of every autistic child. In our program, the laboratory tests we do are expensive, and the treatments rigorous. Some patients drop out of the program for financial reasons. Recently I treated one autistic girl who showed a dramatic 60 percent improvement over the course of a year. Her parents stopped treatment when they heard we needed to do more tests. I felt deeply discouraged. In my experience, based on a limited number of cases, it is unlikely that progress will continue if the patient discontinues therapy before it has been completed. We have found that it is difficult to document 100 percent remissions in our autistic patients, since so few of these children actually continue to the point of having fully completed the program.

Allow me to state this more forcibly. Treatment should not be discontinued when a child appears to be getting better. Ideally, treatment should continue until the biological signs of the dysfunction have disappeared. Some aspects of treatment, such as supporting liver function, may be important over the arc of the child's lifetime. We also have to know when we have cleared the body of the toxic burden, and for this, a second round of laboratory tests may be necessary. The analogy I use is that of a smoldering fire. The residual toxins in the body are like the ashes from a fire that are still smoldering. If you have not put them out completely, you will get a secondary or low-level fire. What was steady upward progress begins to level out, until the child is not progressing any further.

Clearly, the cost of this program is a major challenge that confronts many parents today. Insurance coverage is extremely limited, as is the case for many so-called complementary and alternative therapies. All of this points to the need for a research grant or foundation to help defray costs to the parents of autistic children. As the link between environmental toxins and developmental disorders becomes more widely accepted and understood, I believe more funding will become available for this mind-saving research.

Directives for the Future

Much of the initial funding for what might be called "eco-autism" research will focus on broad-based *prevention* in environmentally sensitive areas. We should look at geographical clusters of autism, such as that found in Brick Township, New Jersey, with an eye toward testing the children themselves for toxic chemicals, rather than merely trying to see whether polluted groundwater correlates with the distribution of autistic cases. For this we will need sophisticated tools sensitive enough to pick up biological and toxicological problems in these children.

The fact that there is a growing body of research and increasing concern about the effects of neurotoxic chemicals on children is a step in the right direction. There is so much that we don't know; many chemicals in the environment have not yet been tested for their possible developmental neurotoxic effects.[2] Recently new attention has been given to how the danger of exposure to certain pesticides is evaluated. According to the 1996 Food Quality Protection Act (FQPA), total exposure of pesticides must pose "no harm" to human health. In particular, according to this legislation, we must take into account the special vulnerability of children, and a chemical's toxicity to children's developing brains and nervous systems; we must consider cumulative exposure at rates higher than to any one individual substance; and exposure via different routes (air, food, water, etc.). This act requires the EPA to determine whether pesticide levels found in food are safe for use in children, taking into account the special vulnerability of children and infants to neurotoxic exposure.

Despite the significant medical advances in the twentieth century, the etiology of the major pediatric diseases remains something of a mystery. In the United States today the most common pediatric diseases are chronic rather than infectious—autism and developmental disorders, asthma, birth defects, child leukemia, and brain cancer. Most of these disorders have dramatically increased in frequency since the 1970s.[3] Exposure to environmental toxins has been posited as one of the major causes of this phenomenon that needs to be explored.

While efforts to prevent autism should receive top priority, let us not forget that millions of children already will have been exposed to xenobiotic chemicals and heavy metals by the time such research begins; some proportion of these children will develop autism. Research focusing on the toxin-removing treatment of autism—the approach laid out in this book—is just as important a scientific mandate as research geared toward prevention.

For decades, our society has been collectively responsible for dumping billions of tons of toxic chemicals into the environment. Now we have an obligation to evaluate and address the effects of these chemicals on children's health. We are living in the midst of a massive experiment, in which the human species is confronted with a toxic burden unlike anything in human history. Children are the unfortunate participants in this experiment, the unwitting subjects who are likely to suffer the greatest harm. We must work together to find ways to protect our children, and our world. We now have the tools within our reach.

Appendix I

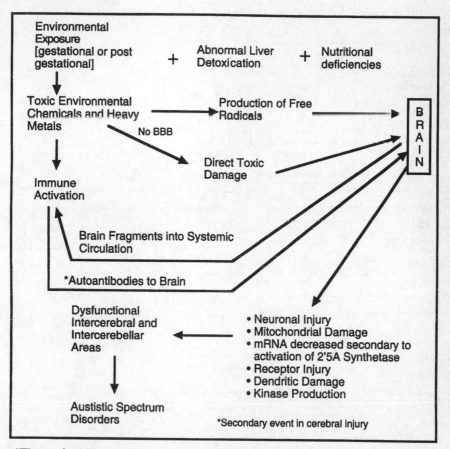

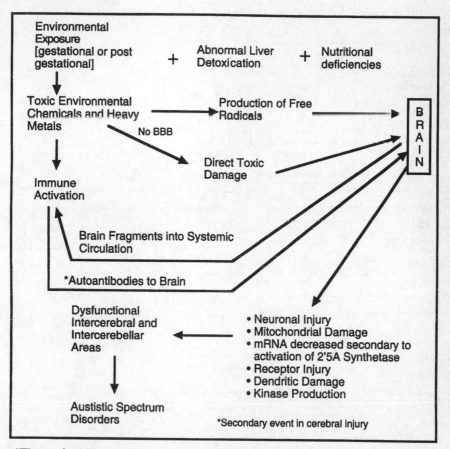

"Theoretical Mechanisms of Neurotoxicity in the Autistic Spectrum Disorders"

This scientific overview of the Edelson theory of autism explains at a glance how environmental toxins, along with a genetic predisposition to poor liver detoxication, can result in injury to the immune system and to the brain. The brain lacks protection in fetal life and early infancy because of the fact that the blood brain barrier is incompletely formed during this period. Toxins can get to the brain leading to injury from the excessive production of free radicals or direct injury to neuronal or interneuronal molecular structures. The immune system is injured leading to an activated system that can cause an autoimmune process attacking brain fragments. This multifaceted illness affects many organs; nonetheless, the brain-related alterations are the most obvious to the casual observer. To the physician with an understanding of clinical molecular medicine, the brain-related effects are just the tip of the autistic iceberg.

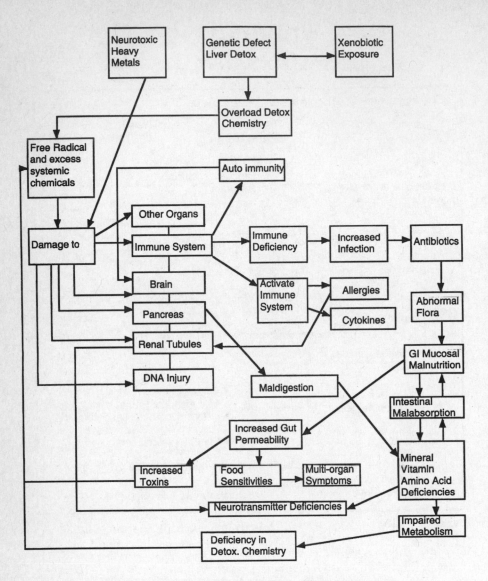

"Autism: A Genetic-Immunotoxicological Syndrome"

The flow chart depicts the convoluted multi-organ systemic illness we call autism. It displays the various connections that lie within the abnormal biology we have studied in these children. Some of the areas of abnormality reveal symptomatic changes in the individual, while others are subclinical and lack any visible or obvious manifestations. A complete understanding of this chart can only be attained by reading about the different aspects of this genetic-immunotoxicological syndrome, as laid out in the book.

Appendix II

An Innovative Approach to the Treatment of Autism
by Stephen B. Edelson, M.D.
Submitted to the new quarterly *Journal of Children's Health*
(for more information, go to:
www.journalofchildrenshealth.org).

Abstract. *Autism is a neurodevelopmental disorder arising from the inter-action of a genetic predisposition and environmental insults during prena-tal life. Based on nutritional, immunological, and toxicological evaluations obtained for over 200 autistic children over the past decade, the author concludes that autistic individuals are born with defective hepatic detoxi-cation, which then predisposes the individual to neurotoxic accumula-tions. Chronic accumulation of xenobiotic and heavy metal neurotoxins, combined with immunotoxicological mechanisms, can result in incremen-tal damage to critical brain structures associated with autism. Appropriate treatment must focus on improving hepatic detoxication, modulating im-mune function, and reducing the overall toxic burden. A series of 15 cases is briefly summarized to help illustrate the merits of this perspective and approach called Edelson Autism Management (EAM). Upon clinical test-ing, all of the patients showed abnormal liver detoxication, as well as other abnormalities such as xenobiotic and heavy metal accumulations, food and chemical allergies, and autoimmune dysfunction. These cases suggest that aggressive reduction of the toxic burden may lead to measur-able reduction in autistic behavior. The series of 15 cases presented here supports the hypothesis that autism has a toxic etiology.*

Introduction

Infantile autism is a behaviorally defined syndrome characterized by patterns of delay and deviance in the development of social, cognitive, and communicative skills.[1] Classical autism is now considered to be part of a spectrum of neurodevelopmental disorders that include Asperger's syn-drome and pervasive developmental disorder not otherwise specified. These three disorders have such a broad range of behavioral consequences in common that they are now considered, collectively, to be part of the broader phenotype of autism known as Autism Spectrum Disorder.[*2] Originally, autism was thought to be caused by parental and social influences, as well as hereditary factors. A growing body of research suggests, however, that chronic exposure to environmental toxins during prenatal and infantile development plays a fundamental role in the pathogenesis of this disorder. Such chronic toxicity becomes amplified in the context of genetic defects in hepatic detoxication mechanisms.[2,3] The author's research, as presented here and elsewhere, suggests that such defects may be universal among autistic children.

Early-life exposures to neurotoxic compounds in the environment are increasingly suspected as playing an etiologic role in autism and other neurodevelopmental disorders.[4,5,6] Both laboratory and epidemiological studies have linked autism with specific exposures or exposure levels. For example, several studies of infants born to women who frequently ingested alcohol during pregnancy found an increased risk of autism.[7,8,9] These studies were relatively small, however, and larger trials are needed to determine the strength of the association. In addition to alcohol, numerous xenobiotics may interfere with the normal ontogeny of developmental processes in the embryonic and newborn nervous system.[10,11,12] The fetal and newborn brains are particularly vulnerable to neurotoxic effects. For example, *in utero* exposure to heavy metals,[13,14] nicotine,[15] and various drugs[16,17] may damage the fetal brain, resulting in neurodevelopmental abnormalities. Additionally, prenatal exposure to pesticides and other synthetic chemicals can further impair the neurobehavioral development of the offspring.[18,19] For example, *in utero* exposure to polychlorinated biphenyls (PCBs) has been associated with lower birth rate and head circumference, as well as other adverse effects, including memory deficits.[20] These chemicals are typically lipophilic and thus are stored in maternal fat before being released into the mother's bloodstream and passed on to the fetus and then to the infant during breastfeeding.[21]

In an earlier paper, Drs. Edelson and Cantor presented the hypothesis that the pathogenesis of autism involves a chronic toxicological mechanism.[22] In that study, all subjects showed abnormal elevations in D-glucaric acid, a catabolite of glucose that is elevated in response to the presence of

---

*Although the narrower term *autistic disorder* is used to refer to classic autism, in this paper I will use the terms *autism* and *autistic* broadly to refer to the larger spectrum of behavioral abnormalities that characterize this group of disorders. Additionally, note that the fourth edition of the *Diagnostic and Statistical Manual of Mental Disorders* (DSM-IV) uses the term *pervasive developmental disorder* (often called *PDD*) to identify this broader grouping of disorders.

foreign chemicals. Chronic exposure to toxic xenobiotics can trigger hepatic enzyme activities that lead to the formation of D-glucaric acid. Thus, the data from that study seemed to confirm the author's hypothesis. We subsequently examined more than 70 autistic children, and found that all 70 had abnormal liver detoxication and all showed abnormally high levels of toxic chemicals in their tissues; a large percentage also showed high concentrations of heavy metals.[23]

Based on the author's clinical observations over the past decade, autistic disorders represent the final expression of a toxic etiology that may be unique to our postindustrial era. Appropriate treatment must attempt to normalize the biochemical and toxicological profile of the autistic individual, as this profile appears to be integral to the pathogenesis and progression of this disorder. A series of cases are briefly described to help illustrate the efficacy of therapeutic strategies the author has found effective in his Atlanta-based environmental medicine clinic. This approach called Edelson Autism Management (EAM) evolved over the past decade in the course of analyzing blood and tissue specimens from autistic children, then correlating these data with behavioral data obtained before and after treatment. The approach is designed to improve or reverse the underlying metabolic abnormalities that afflict autistic individuals through nutritional pharmacology, detoxication and immunologic modulation, and other noninvasive strategies that are part of environmental medicine.[24]

A Series of Cases from the Atlanta Clinic

Toxicological and immunological profiles were obtained for 15 autistic children, along with outcome measures based on scores from the Autism Treatment Evaluation Checklist (ATEC). This instrument, a product of the Autism Research Institute, was specifically designed to evaluate the effectiveness of various treatments for autistic individuals. The ATEC entails a simple Internet-based scoring procedure that requires the parents, guardians, or caregivers to fill out an evaluation of their child's behavioral and mental capacities. The instrument calculates subscale scores and a summary score, and each score is weighted according to the response and the corresponding subscale. The higher the subscale scores (and thus the total score), the greater the severity of autistic impairment. Changes in total score are reported as percentages that indicate the extent of improvement between the most recent evaluation and the initial baseline evaluation.

Case 1 (SM). This female patient showed very high levels of mercury, as well as elevated lead and tin. Her main behavioral symptom was having tantrums throughout the day. Additionally, her liver detoxication tests showed elevated phase I activity, which is conducive to oxidative stress. Other findings of interest included high urinary mercapturic acid levels, indicating chemical toxicity; low zinc and manganese levels, both common in autistic children and probably linked with poor antioxidant capacity; elevated copper levels, which is consistent with oxidative stress; leaky gut (breach of intestinal lining), resulting in excessive absorption of food and microbial antigens; candida overgrowth; blastocystis hominis (parasitic infection); maldigestion and malabsorption; multiple food allergies, including IgA positive tests for both gluten and casein (which may have led to the leaky gut); and allergies to inhalants. Within a period of six months following completion of chelation, sauna therapy, antifungal therapy, and other EAM strategies, she began to talk (she had been nonverbal) and her tantrums stopped. Six years after initiation of therapy, ATEC scores indicate that she is functioning at a 95 percent level (100% being normal). She is attending prep school and, with the exception of occasional anxiety, is considered normal.

Case 2 (SJ). This male patient showed high blood levels of two common xenobiotics, hexane and methyl pentane, as well as high levels of only one heavy metal, tin. His mineral levels (zinc, magnesium, and potassium) were low. The liver detoxication parameters were abnormal, with elevated phase I and low phase II, as well as glutathione deficiency. This can be due either to genetic defects, or to excessive exposure to toxins in the blood; both can cause phase I to be upregulated. A yeast overgrowth was also indicated, along with infection by pseudomonas, a pathogenic bacteria; this is consistent with the observed intestinal malabsorption. The patient also showed high levels of oxidative stress, as indicated by increased lipid peroxidation. Nearly all of these children show high oxidative stress levels, which may play a critical role in neurotoxicity. The patient showed marked improvement in most of his behavioral parameters within six months. Eleven months from the inception of therapy, this patient has shown a 64 percent improvement based on ATEC scores.

Case 3 (HT). This male patient showed elevated levels of toxic xenobiotics (benzene and styrene) as well as an array of heavy metal elevations, including lead, aluminum, arsenic, cobalt, nickel, tin, and titanium. He also had a severe autoimmune dysfunction, with elevated antibodies to

MAG protein, oligodendrocyte, and capillary endothelial cell. These constitute three major sources of neurotoxicity: chemicals, metals, and autoimmunity. Additionally, he showed abnormal liver detoxication, excessive oxidative stress, candida overgrowth, maldigestion, renal tubular injury, and a low secretory IgA in the intestine resulting in increased intestinal pathogens (group D enterococcus). After one year of completing therapy, the ATEC test results indicate that the patient has improved by approximately 76 percent.

Case 4 (RW). This male patient showed elevations in styrene (a xenobiotic), lead, aluminum, nickel, and titanium. Abnormal liver detoxication manifested as decreased phase I and high phase II activities, ostensibly in response to the toxins. Cysteine, sulfate, and glutathione were all decreased, consistent with genetic defects and nutritional issues. Autoimmune dysfunction was indicated by antibodies to tubulin and myelin protein. Gastrointestinal studies revealed low secretory IgA, along with colonic inflammation and low chymotrypsin levels. Food and inhalant allergies were also present. He was significantly autistic. One year following the initiation of treatment (he still comes in for weakly chelation), this child is taking violin lessons. The patient showed a 53 percent improvement 14 months from the inception of therapy.

Case 5 (PB). This male patient showed massive accumulations of heavy metals, including lead, aluminum, tin, nickel, cobalt, gallium, titanium, and rubidium. Organophosphorous pesticide levels were also high. (These pesticides are commonly sprayed in homes, shopping malls, and schools.) He also showed signs of toluene toxicity, abnormal liver detoxication (elevated phase I, low phase II), and significant autoimmunity. Also present in this boy were the following: severe oxidative stress, *Candida albicans* overgrowth, leaky gut, and allergies to gluten and casein. Allergies to other foods, as well as inhalants, were present. A 54 percent improvement was evident seven months after the initiation of therapy.

Case 6 (HA). This female patient showed severe heavy metal toxicity, again without mercury. The metals that were elevated included lead, cobalt, nickel, tin, titanium, with slight elevations in tungsten, gallium, and aluminum. Conversely, levels of copper, manganese, and magnesium were deficient. A number of pesticide residues were also found to be elevated, and xylene was present in the urine. She also showed high levels of oxidative stress, DNA injury, malabsorption, and maldigestion. Detoxication tests showed a genetic defect in sulfoxidation (phase I, lacking the sulfite oxidase enzyme), while phase II was extremely high, indicating that the liver was apparently overactive in eliminating toxins. Allergies to foods and inhalants were also present. The patient showed a 49 percent improvement over a five-month period.

Case 7 (FI). This male patient showed massive chemical and heavy metal overload. The heavy metals did not include mercury, but did include aluminum, lead, nickel, and tin, among others. He had clear evidence of oxidative stress with DNA injury. His liver detoxication abnormalities were indicated by low glutathione and sulfate oxidase enzyme activity. Also present were candidiasis and intestinal maldigestion, along with allergies to food and inhalants. A 77 percent improvement was reported one year from the initiation of therapy.

Case 8 (GSK). This male patient showed heavy accumulations of toxic chemicals (styrene, hexane, and methyl pentanes), as well as clear problems with liver detoxication, including low phase II activity. Malabsorption and oxidative stress were also present, as were low levels of several minerals (zinc, molybdenum, and manganese). A 63 percent improvement was noted 14 months from the initiation of therapy. However, the parents discontinued the EAM program after 10 months prior to the final evaluation, so the therapeutic improvement plateaued. This is a common occurrence with parents who assume that the child will continue to show improvement after the initial series of treatments; unfortunately, unless treatments are completed, the improvement invariably levels off.

Case 9 (DN). This male patient showed evidence of chemical overload, as indicated by high levels of styrene, dichloromethane, hexane, and methyl pentane. Elevations in several metals (tin, lead, and mercury) were also evident. He showed abnormal liver detoxication, as indicated by high phase I and high phase II activity. Lipid peroxide levels were also high, indicating oxidative stress. Also present were maldigestion, nutritional deficiencies (potassium, zinc, and magnesium), food and inhalant allergies, and high levels of cadmium in the blood, which did not show up in the urinary analysis. (This may have been an acute exposure. Seven months after initiation of therapy, the patient showed an 86 percent improvement in behavioral variables.)

Case 10 (AN). This male patient showed high levels of various toxic chemicals (endrin, trimethyl benzene, 2-methylpentane, and hexane) as well as high levels of lead, tin, and mercury. Also present were oxidative stress, oxidative DNA damage, maldigestion, nutritional deficiencies (magnesium, zinc, and selenium), food and inhalant allergies, candida overgrowth, intestinal parasites, and autoimmune problems (antibodies to myelin). Aberrant liver detoxication was indicated by increased phase I activity and decreased phase II activity, along with low glutathione levels. He improved to the 90th percentile. An 88 percent improvement was reported approximately four years from the initial baseline evaluation.

Case 11 (BC). This female patient had high concentrations of organophosphorous pesticides as well as heavy metal overload (lead, tin, and mercury). Abnormal liver detoxication was indicated by low sulfate oxidase activity and decreased phase II activity. Tests revealed evidence of oxidative stress, oxidative DNA damage, nutritional deficiencies (potassium and selenium), leaky gut, food and inhalant allergies, candida overgrowth, and autoimmune problems (antibodies to brain endothelial cells). She also showed poor pancreatic function and hypochlorhydria, both contributing to severe maldigestion. She has shown a 72 percent improvement in two years. (Anything over 70 percent often appears to be normal; anxiety, sleep problems, and other minor complaints may still be present.)

Case 12 (GJ). This female patient showed massive chemical and heavy metal toxicity. Xenobiotic elevations included styrene, mirex, toluene, xylene, DDT, tetrachlorehylene, and dichloromethane. Metal elevations included tin, lead, cadmium, and mercury. Also present were leaky gut, malabsorption, candida overgrowth, food and inhalant allergies, mineral deficiencies (zinc, molybdenum, potassium), aberrant liver detoxication (high phase I, high phase II, low sulfate oxidase and glutathione), and high oxidative stress levels. The parents were unable to have their child undergo the full EAM program for various reasons, so therapy was sporadic over a four-year period. Despite the lack of consistent therapy, a 66 percent improvement was reported.

Case 13 (ST). This male patient showed high levels of toluene and organophosphates, as well as heavy metal overload involving lead, mercury, aluminum, arsenic, nickel, and tin. Liver detoxication was abnormal, with low phase II, low glutathione, superoxide dismutase, and sulfate oxidase. Maldigestion, food and inhalant allergies, and oxidative stress were also present. We have worked with him only a short time. This is an older child (nine years old upon entering clinic, in contrast to most children, who come in between three and five years of age). ATEC scores indicated a 35 percent improvement six months from the initiation of therapy.

Case 14 (BC). This male patient showed high levels of lead, benzene, xylene, ethylbenzene, and styrene. Oxidative stress was quite pronounced, as indicated by low glutathione levels and high levels of hydroxyl radicals, lipid peroxide, hydroperoxide, and oxidized DNA damage. Liver detoxication was abnormal, as indicated by high phase I and high phase II enzyme activities. Also present were food and inhalant allergies, leaky gut, low chymotrypsin levels, and maldigestion. A 47 percent improvement was recorded one year from the inception of therapy.

Case 15 (RLA).   This male patient showed evidence of heavy metal overload, based on high levels of mercury, lead, nickel, and aluminum. Autoimmune dysfunction was indicated by antibodies to tubulin, myelin basic protein, and several other neuronal proteins. Also present were the following: elevated oxidative stress, maldigestion, food and inhalant allergies, leaky gut, low intestinal secretory IgA, and elevations in both phase I and phase II liver enzymes. Before and after testing the patient showed a 100 percent improvement one year from the initiation of therapy. Independent evaluation by a neuropsychologist indicates that this child is now functioning normally for his age in all respects.

Discussion and Conclusion

All 15 of these children showed evidence of substantial xenobiotic and heavy metal burden. This suggests that a toxic etiology underlies the cerebral dysfunction that governs autistic behavior. The 15 cases are typical of those that have been biochemically evaluated by the author over the past decade. In addition to the xenobiotic and/or heavy metal exposures, several other common themes are apparent in these cases, including abnormal genetic liver detoxication, oxidative stress, autoimmune dysfunction, gastrointestinal abnormalities, candida overgrowth, and food and inhalant allergies. Aberrant genetics in liver detoxication characteristics were identified in a number of patients.

This case series extends previously reported evidence by the author that autistic individuals suffer from neurodevelopmental damage that likely arises from an interaction between toxic environmental factors, defective hepatic detoxication, immunologic dysfunction, and oxidative damage to neural tissues. These factors may coalesce to promote chronic neurotoxicity and, consequently, the pathological alterations of neurological structures that characterize the development of autism. Toxic metals and chemicals lead to increased oxidative stress, which then results in molecular neuronal injury and neurobehavioral dysfunction.

In a previous case series report (n=20) by this author, it was noted that

100 percent of the cases showed aberrant liver detoxication profiles.[25] Sixteen out of eighteen autistic children whose blood analyses were available showed evidence of levels of toxic chemicals exceeding adult maximum tolerance. Although any one case series can only aid in the formulation of a new hypothesis, such studies still represent an important interface between clinical medicine and epidemiology. The interpretability of the data is limited by the lack of an appropriate comparison group. It is possible that an association may be suggested here where none actually exists, or that an alternate causal relationship is entirely obscured. For these reasons, a case series cannot be used to test the presence of a statistical association. Rigorous data from analytic studies are now needed to substantiate the author's hypothesis, which has strong biological plausibility.

Another limitation of this study is the use of the ATEC instrument without independent evaluations being conducted by a trained developmental psychiatrist or neurodevelopmental pediatrician. Ideally, all cases would have a comprehensive, independent evaluation to confirm the ATEC findings, as occurred with the last case report (#15). It is possible that mothers would tend to record more favorable scores over time. Given the rigorous demands of the program, along with the parents' desire to have their children improve, one might speculate that parents may tend to exaggerate the improvements they have seen in their children. However, even if we assume that such bias clearly exists, and that it would skew the outcome data considerably (even by as much as 10 to 20 percent), the improvements seen in most of these children remain compelling.

Despite the rigorous demands placed on parents and children when they undergo the EAM protocols, it is also true that the program can be immensely rewarding. By attending to the underlying problems of abnormal liver detoxication, food and chemical allergies, and toxic metal and chemical exposures, a sizable neurotoxic burden can be removed from the autistic body, and this may facilitate recovery in these children. Using the ATEC questionnaire, based on over 200 cases studied to date, the average stated improvement in our patients after approximately two years of treatment is 61 percent. Many parents are astonished at how rapidly their children begin to make progress in developing verbal and social skills following the initiation of detoxification therapy.

In summary, the cases presented here support the author's hypothesis that a toxic etiology underlies autistic spectrum disorders. Abnormal liver detoxication, perhaps caused by genetic insult prior to conception, may play a pivotal role in the progressive course of autism. With the help of intensive detoxification, chelation, immune modulation, and nutritional therapy, children attending the Atlanta-based clinic have shown significant improvement in autistic symptoms. These treatments do not cause harm, and they appear to be more effective for children under five years of age. The EAM program reflects a growing trend in environmental medicine that focuses on the underlying cellular and molecular factors intrinsic to the pathogenesis of neurodevelopmental disorders. Clinical trials are now needed to test the efficacy of this multifaceted therapeutic approach to targeting the neurotoxic physiology of autism.

References

Chapter 1

1. Gent TV, Heijnen CJ, Treffers PD. Autism and the immune system. Journal of Child Psychology & Psychiatry & Allied Disciplines. 38(3):337–49, 1997.
2. Bland JS. Neurobiochemistry: a new paradigm for managing brain biochemical disturbances. Journal of Orthomolecular Medicine. 9(3):177–85, 1994.
3. Ananth J et al. Hepatic diseases and psychiatric illness: relationships and treatment. Psychotherapy & Psychosomatics. 62:146–59, 1994.
4. Bland JS, Bralley JA. Nutritional upregulation of hepatic detoxification enzymes. Journal of Applied Nutrition. 44(3&4), 1992.
5. Waring RH. Enzyme and sulfur oxidation deficiencies in autistic children with known food and chemical intolerances. Journal of Orthomolecular Medicine. 8(4), 1993.
6. Edelson SB, Cantor DS. Autism: xenobiotic influences. Toxicology & Industrial Health. 14(4):553–63, 1998.
7. Talalay P, Prochaska HJ, Spencer SR. Regulation of enzymes that detoxify the electrophilic forms of chemical carcinogens. Princess Takamatsu Symposia. 21:177–87, 1990.
8. Prochaska HJ, Santamaria AB, Talalay P. Rapid detection of inducers of enzymes that protect against carcinogens. Proceedings of the National Academy of Sciences of the United States of America. 89(6):2394–98, 1992.
9. Edelson SB, Cantor DS. 1998. Op cit.
10. Comi AM, Zimmerman AW, Frye VH, Law PA, Peeden JN. Familial clus-

tering of autoimmune disorders and evaluation of medical risk factors in autism. Journal of Child Neurology. 14(6):388–94, 1999.

11. Sakic B, Szechtman H, Denburg JA. Neurobehavioral alterations in auto-immune mice. Neuroscience & Biobehavioral Reviews. 21(3):327–40, 1997.

12. Grant EC, Howard JM, Davies S, Chasty H, et al. Zinc deficiency in children with dyslexia: concentrations of zinc and other minerals in sweat and hair. British Medical Journal. 296(6622): 607–9, 1988.

13. Egger J, Carter CM, Graham PJ, Gumley D, Soothill JF. Controlled trial of oligoantigenic treatment in the hyperkinetic syndrome. Lancet 1(8428): 540–45, 1985.

14. Pfeiffer CC, Braverman ER. Zinc, the brain and behavior. Biological Psychiatry. 17(4):513–32, 1982.

15. Barlow PJ, Sidani SA. Metal imbalance and hyperactivity. Acta Pharmaceutrca & Pharmacology. 59(Suppl 7): 458–62. 1986.

16. Wecker L, Miller SB, Cochran SR, Dugger DL, Johnson WD. Trace element concentrations in hair from autistic children. Journal of Mental Deficiency Research. 29 (Pt 1):15–22, 1985.

17. Wang FD, Bian W, Kong LW, Zhao FJ, Guo JS, Jing NH. Maternal zinc deficiency impairs brain nestin expression in prenatal and postnatal mice. Cell Research. 11(2):135–41, 2001.

18. Bhatnagar S, Taneja S. Zinc and cognitive development. British Journal of Nutrition. 85 Suppl 2:S139–45, 2001.

19. Johnson S. Micronutrient accumulation and depletion in schizophrenia, epilepsy, autism and Parkinson's disease? Medical Hypotheses. 56(5): 641–45, 2001.

Chapter 2

1. Edelson SB, Cantor DS. Autism: xenobiotic influences. Toxicology & Industrial Health. 14(4):553–63, 1998.

2. American Psychiatric Association, DSM-IV, 2000.

3. Bhaumik S, Branford D, McGrother C, Thorp C. Autistic traits in adults with learning disabilities. British Journal of Psychiatry. 170:502–6, 1997.

4. Myhr G. Autism and other pervasive developmental disorders: exploring the dimensional view. Canadian Journal of Psychiatry—Revue Canadienne de Psychiatrie. 43(6):589–95, 1998.

5. Ruhl D, Bolte S, Poustka F. Speech development and intelligence in autism: how uniform is Asperger's syndrome. Nervenarzt. 72(7):535–40. 2001.

6. Lainhart JE, Piven J. Diagnosis, treatment, and neurobiology of autism in children. [Review] Current Opinion in Pediatrics. 7(4):392–400, 1995.

7. Piven J, Palmer P, Landa R, Santangelo S, Jacobi D, Childress D. Personality and language characteristics in parents from multiple-incidence

autism families. American Journal of Medical Genetics. 74(4):398–411, 1997.

8. Piven J, Palmer P. Cognitive deficits in parents from multiple-incidence autism families. Journal of Child Psychology & Psychiatry & Allied Disciplines. 38(8):1011–21, 1997.

9. Piven J, Palmer P, Jacobi D, Childress D, Arndt S. Broader autism phenotype: evidence from a family history study of multiple-incidence autism families. American Journal of Psychiatry. 154(2):185–90, 1997.

10. Rapin I, Dunn M. Language disorders in children with autism. [Review] Seminars in Pediatric Neurology. 4(2):86–92, 1997.

11. Accardo P, Whitman B. Toe walking. A marker for language disorders in the developmentally disabled. Clinical Pediatrics. 28(8):347–50, 1989.

12. Rogers SJ, DiLalla DL. Age of symptom onset in young children with pervasive developmental disorders. Journal of the American Academy of Child & Adolescent Psychiatry. 29(6):863–72, 1990.

13. Rogers SJ, DiLalla DL. Age of symptom onset in young children with pervasive developmental disorders. Journal of the American Academy of Child & Adolescent Psychiatry. 29(6):863–72, 1990.

14. Baron-Cohen S, Wheelwright S, Skinner R, Martin J, Clubley E. The autism spectrum quotient. Journal of Autism and Developmental Disorders 31(1):5–17, 2001.

15. Dennis M, Lazenby AL, Lockyer L. Inferential language in high functioning children with autism. Journal of Autism and Developmental Disorders 31(1):47–54. 2001.

16. Restall G, Magill-Evans J. Play and preschool children with autism. American Journal of Occupational Therapy. 48(2):113–20, 1994.

17. Meltz BF. Boston Globe. FEAT Newsletter. March 29, 2001.

18. Cowley G. Understanding Autism. Newsweek, p. 48. July 31, 2000.

19. Schafer L, Editorial. FEAT Daily Newsletter. July 10, 2001.

20. Rinehart NJ, Bradshaw JL, Brereton AV, Tonge BJ. Journal of Autism and Developmental Disorders. 31(1):79–88, 2001.

21. Beversdorf DQ, Anderson JM, Manning SE, Anderson SL, Nordgren RE, Felopulos GJ, Bauman ML. Journal of Autism and Developmental Disorders. 31(1):97–101, 2001.

22. Kelly SJ, Macaruso P, Sokol SM. Mental calculation in an autistic savant: a case study. Journal of Clinical & Experimental Neuropsychology. 19(2): 172–84, 1997.

23. Dowker A, Hermelin B, Pring L. A savant poet. Psychological Medicine. 26(5):913–24, 1996.

24. Snyder AW, Thomas M. Autistic artists give clues to cognition. Perception. 26(1):93–96, 1997.

25. Cowley G. 2000. Op cit. p. 50.

26. Gadow KD. An overview of three decades of research in pediatric psychopharmacoepidemiology. Journal of Child & Adolescent Psychopharmacology. 7(4):219–36, 1997.

27. Warren RP, Singh VK. Elevated serotonin levels in autism: association with the major histocompatibility complex. Neuropsychobiology. 34(2): 72–5, 1996.

28. Cook EH, Leventhal BL. The serotonin system in autism. Current Opinion in Pediatrics. 8(4):348–54, 1996.

29. Levine J, Aviram A, Holan A, Ring A, Barak Y, Belmaker RH. Inositol treatment of autism. Journal of Neural Transmission. 104(2–3):307–10, 1997.

30. Cook EH, Leventhal BL. The serotonin system in autism. Current Opinion in Pediatrics. 8(4):348–54, 1996.

31. McDougle CJ, Naylor ST, Cohen DJ, Aghajanian GK, Heninger GR, Price LH. Effects of tryptophan depletion in drug-free adults with autistic disorder. Archives of General Psychiatry. 53(11):993–1000, 1996.

32. Sloman L. Use of medication in pervasive developmental disorders. Psychiatric Clinics of North America. 14(1):165–82, 1991.

33. Steingard RJ, Zimnitzky B, DeMaso DR, Bauman ML, Bucci JP. Sertraline treatment of transition-associated anxiety and agitation in children with autistic disorder. Journal of Child and Adolescent Psychopharmacology. 7(1):9–15, 1997.

34. Linday LA. Oral famotidine: a potential treatment for children with autism. Medical Hypotheses. 48(5):381–86, 1997.

35. Hatch-Rasmussen C. Sensory integration. Autism Research Institute. 2000.

36. Rimland B, Edelson SM. Pilot study of auditory integration training on autism. Journal of Autism and Development Disorders. 25:61–70, 1995.

37. Kezuka E. The role of touch in facilitated communication. Journal of Autism & Developmental Disorders. 27(5):571–93, 1997.

38. Lightdale JR, Heyman MB. Secretin: cure or snake oil for autism in the new millennium? Journal of Pediatric Gastroenterology & Nutrition. 29(2):114–15, 1999.

39. Owley T, Steele E, Corsello C, Risi S, et al. A double-blind, placebo-controlled trial of secretin for the treatment of autistic disorder. Medscape General Medicine. E2. October 6, 1999.

40. Dolske MC, Spollen J, McKay S, Lancashire E, Tolbert L. A preliminary trial of ascorbic acid as supplemental therapy for autism. Progress in Neuro-Psychopharmacology & Biological Psychiatry. 17(5):765–74, 1993.

41. Jan JE, O'Donnell ME. Use of melatonin in the treatment of pediatric sleep disorders. Journal of Pineal Research. 21(4): 193–99. 1996

42. Freeman BJ. Guidelines for evaluating intervention programs for children

with autism. Journal of Autism & Developmental Disorders. 27(6):641–51, 1997.

43. Courchesne E. Brainstem, cerebellar, and limbic neuroanatomical abnormalities in autism. Current Opinion in Neurobiology. 7(2): 269–78, 1997.

44. Baron-Cohen S, Allen J, Gillberg C. Can autism be detected at 18 months? The needle, the haystack, and the CHAT. British Journal of Psychiatry. 161:839–43, 1992.

45. Teitelbaum P, Teitelbaum O, Nye J, Freeman J, Maurer RG. Movement analysis in infancy may be useful for early diagnosis of autism. Proceedings of the National Academy of Sciences, USA, 95: 13982–87, 1998.

46. Johnson MH, Siddons F, Frith U, Morton J. Can autism be predicted on the basis of infant screening tests? Developmental Medicine & Child Neurology. 34(4):316–20, 1992.

47. Mars AE, Mauk JE, Dowrick PW. Symptoms of pervasive developmental disorders as observed in prediagnostic home videos of infants and toddlers. Journal of Pediatrics. 132(3 Pt 1):500–4, 1998.

48. Cowley G. 2000. Op cit. p 51.

Chapter 3

1. Cowley G. Understanding autism. Newsweek, p. 48. July 31, 2000.

2. Bryson SE, Smith IM. Epidemiology of autism: prevalence, associated characteristics, and service delivery. Mental Retardation and Developmental Disabilities Research Reviews, 4: 97–103, 1998.

3. Vaccine Fact Sheets: Autism Prevalence. National Vaccine Program Office. U.S. Centers for Disease Control and Prevention, Atlanta, Georgia. Website: http://www.cdc.gov/ncbddd/dd/ddautism.htm. 2001.

4. Vaccine Fact Sheets: Autism Prevalence. 2001. Ibid.

5. Connor T. What's causing autism rise? New York Post, October 10, 2000.

6. Fombonne E. Is there an epidemic of autism? Pediatrics. 107(2):411–12, 2001.

7. Rapin I. An 8-year-old boy with autism. JAMA. 285(13):1749–57, 2001.

8. DeFrancesco L. Scientists question rise in autism. Nature Medicine 7(6):645, 2001.

9. Lemasters GK, Perreault SD, Hales BF, Hatch M, et al. Workshop to identify critical windows of exposure for children's health: reproductive health in children and adolescents work group summary. Environmental Health Perspectives.108 Suppl 3:505–9, 2000.

10. Rice D, Barone S. Critical periods of vulnerability for the developing nervous system: evidence from humans and animal models. Environmental Health Perspectives. 108 Suppl 3:511–33, 2000.

11. Goldman LR, Koduru S. Chemicals in the environment and developmental toxicity to children: a public health and policy perspective. Environmental Health Perspectives. 108 Suppl 3:443–48, 2000.

12. Myers GJ, Davidson PW. Prenatal methylmercury exposure and children: neurologic, developmental, and behavioral research. Environmental Health Perspectives. 106 Suppl 3:841–7, 1998.

13. Baraldi M, Zanoli P, Rossi T, Borella P, Caselgrandi E, Petraglia F. Neurobehavioral and neurochemical abnormalities of pre- and postnatally lead-exposed rats: zinc, copper and calcium status. Neurobehavioral Toxicology & Teratology. 7(5):499–509, 1985.

14. Weiss B, Landrigan PJ. The developing brain and the environment. Environmental Health Perspectives Supplement. 108(3):373–74, 2000.

15. Ernst M, Moolchan ET, Robinson ML. Behavioral and neural consequences of prenatal exposure to nicotine. Journal of the American Academy of Child & Adolescent Psychiatry. 40(6):630–41, 2001.

16. Nulman I, Rovet J, Greenbaum R, Loebstein M, Wolpin J, Pace-Asciak P, Koren G. Neurodevelopment of adopted children exposed in utero to cocaine: the Toronto Adoption Study. Clinical & Investigative Medicine— Medecine Clinique et Experimentale. 24(3):129–37, 2001.

17. Budden SS. Intrauterine exposure to drugs and alcohol: how do the children fare? Medscape Womens Health. 1(10):6, 1996.

18. Chambers JE, Levi PE, ed. Organophosphates, chemistry, fate, and effects. San Diego, CA: Academic Press; 1992.

19. Arlien-Soberg P. Solvent neurotoxicity. Boca Raton, FL: CRC Press; 1992.

20. Cowley, G. Understanding autism. Newsweek, p. 52. July 31, 2000.

21. Bertrand J, Mars A, Boyle C, Bove F, Yeargin-Allsopp M. Prevalence of autism in a United States population: Brick Township, NJ. Paediatric & Perinatal Epidemiology. 15(4):A4, 2001.

22. Boorman GA. Drinking water disinfection byproducts: review and approach to toxicity evaluation. Environmental Health Perspectives. 107 Suppl 1:207–17, 1999.

23. Public Health Assessment, Brick Township Investigation (a/k/a Brick Township Autism Investigation. Superfund Site Assessment Branch, Division of Health Assessment and Consultation Agency for Toxic Substances and Disease Registry. 2000.

24. Bove FJ, Fulcomer MC, Klotz JB, Esmart J, Dufficy EM, Savrin JE. Public drinking water contamination and birth outcomes. American Journal of Epidemiology. 141(9):850–62, 1995.

25. Dodds L, King WD. Relation between trihalomethane compounds and birth defects. Occupational & Environmental Medicine. 58(7):443–46, 2001.

26. Klotz JB, Pyrch LA. Neural tube defects and drinking water disinfection by-products. Epidemiology. 10:383–90, 1999.

27. Rodier PM. The early origins of autism. Scientific American. 282(2):56–63, 2000.

28. Rodier PM, Ingram JL, Tisdale B, Nelson S, Romano J. Embryological origin for autism: developmental anomalies of the cranial nerve motor nuclei. Journal of Comparative Neurology. 370(2):247–61, 1996.

29. Ingram JL, Peckham SM, Tisdale B, Rodier PM. Prenatal exposure of rats to valproic acid reproduces the cerebellar anomalies associated with autism. Neurotoxicology & Teratology. 22(3):319–24, 2000.

30. Brennan RJ, Schiestl RH. Chloroform and carbon tetrachloride induce intrachromosomal recombination and oxidative free radicals in Saccharomyces cerevisiae. Mutation Research. 397(2):271–78, 1998.

31. Dodds L, King WD. 2001. Op cit.

32. Dodds L, King W, Woolcott C, Pole J. Trihalomethanes in public water supplies and adverse birth outcomes. Epidemiology. 10(3):233–37, 1999.

33. Halsey CL, Collin MF, Anderson CL. Extremely low-birth-weight children and their peers. A comparison of school-age outcomes. Archives of Pediatrics & Adolescent Medicine. 150(8):790–94, 1996.

34. Kramer MD, Lynch CF, Isacson P, Hanson JW. The association of waterborne chloroform with intrauterine growth retardation. Epidemiology. 3(5):407–13, 1992.

35. Bove FJ, Fulcomer MC, Klotz JB, Esmart J, Dufficy EM, Savrin JE. Public drinking water contamination and birth outcomes. American Journal of Epidemiology. 141(9):850–62, 1995.

36. Waller K, Swan SH, DeLorenze G, Hopkins B. Trihalomethanes in drinking water and spontaneous abortion. Epidemiology. 9(2):134–40, 1998.

37. Gallagher MD, Nuckols JR, Stallones L, Savitz DA. Exposure to trihalomethanes and adverse pregnancy outcomes. Epidemiology. 9(5):484–89, 1998.

38. Balster RL, Borzelleca JF. Behavioral toxicity of trihalomethane contaminants of drinking water in mice. Environmental Health Perspectives. 46:127–36, 1982.

39. Lilly PD, Ross TM, Pegram RA. Trihalomethane comparative toxicity: acute renal and hepatic toxicity of chloroform and bromodichloromethane following aqueous gavage. Fundamental & Applied Toxicology. 40(1):101–10, 1997.

40. Foster KR, Vecchia P, Repacholi MH. Risk management: science and the precautionary principle. Science. 288(5468):979–81, 2000.

41. Edelson SB, Cantor DS. Autism: xenobiotic influences. Toxicology & Industrial Health. 14(4):553–63, 1998.

42. Kaplan S, Morris, J. Kids at Risk. U.S. News & World Report, June 19, 2000.

43. Landrigan PJ, Carlson JE, Bearer CF, Cranmer JS, Bullard RD, Etzel RA,

Groopman J, McLachlan JA, Perera FP, Reigart JR, Robison L, Schell L, Suk WA. Children's health and the environment: a new agenda for prevention research. Environmental Health Perspectives. 106 Suppl 3:787–94, 1998.

44. Weiss B, Landrigan PJ. The developing brain and the environment: an introduction. Environmental Health Perspectives. 108 Suppl 3:373–4, 2000.

45. Liu G, Elsner J. Review of the multiple chemical exposure factors which may disturb human behavioral development. Sozial- und Praventivmedizin. 40(4):209–17, 1995.

46. Needleman HL. Behavioral toxicology. Environmental Health Perspectives. 103 Suppl 6:77–79, 1995.

47. Niswander KR, Gordon M. The women and their pregnancies. U.S. Government Printing Office. DHEW Pub. No. 73–379. Washington, D.C. 1972.

48. Felicetti T. Parents of autistic children: some notes on a chemical connection. Milieu Therapy. 1:13–16, 1981.

49. Bearer C. How are children different from adults? Environmental Health Perspectives, 103 (Supp 6), 1995.

50. Gillberg C. Brief report: onset at age 14 of a typical autistic syndrome. A case report of a girl with herpes simplex encephalitis. Journal of Autism and Developmental Disorders, 16:369–75, 1986.

51. Barton M, Volkmar F. How commonly are known medical conditions associated with autism? Journal of Autism & Developmental Disorders. 28(4):273–78, 1998.

52. Bartholome K, Byrd DJ, Kaufman S, Milstein S. Atypical phenylketonuria with normal phenylalanine hydroxylase and dihydropteridine reductase activity in vitro. Pediatrics, 59:757–61, 1977.

53. Chen CH, Hsiao KJ. A Chinese classic phenylketonuria manifested as autism. British Journal of Psychiatry, 155:251–53, 1989.

54. Friedman E. The autistic syndrome and phenylketonuria. Schizophrenia, 1:249–61, 1969.

55. Kotsopoulos S, Kutty KM. Histidinemia and infantile autism. Journal of Autism and Developmental Disorders, 11:271–83, 1981.

56. Shih VE, Madigan PM. Routine newborn screenings of histidinemia. New England Journal of Medicine, 291:1214–19, 1974.

57. Duran M, Beemer FA, Van de Heiden C, Korteland J, de Bree PK, Brink M, Wadman SK. Combined deficiency of xanthine oxidase and sulfite oxidase. A defect of molybdenum metabolism or transport? Journal of Inherited Metabolic Disease, 1:175–78, 1978.

58. Hunt A, Dennis J. Psychiatric disorders among children with tuberous sclerosis. Developmental Medicine and Child Neurology. 29:190–98, 1987.

59. Cantu ES, Stone JW, Wing AA, Langee HR, Williams CA. Cytogenic survey for autistic fragile-X carriers in a mental retardation center. American Journal of Mental Retardation, 94:442–47, 1990.

60. Cohen IL, Vietze PM, Sudhalter V, Jenkins ED, Brown WT. Effects of age and communication level on eye contact in fragile X males and non-fragile X autistic males. American Journal of Medical Genetics, 38:498–502, 1991.

61. Chess S. Follow-up report on autism in congenital rubella. Journal of Autism and Childhood Schizophrenia, 7:68–81, 1977.

62. Desmond MM, Wilson GS, Melnick JL, Singer DB, Zion TE, Rudolph AJ, Pineda RG, Ziai MH, Blattney RJ. Congenital rubella encephalitis. Journal of Pediatrics, 71:311–31, 1967.

63. Ahlfors K, Ivarsson SA, Harris S, Svanberg L, Holmqvist R, Lernmakr B, Theander G. Congenital cytomegalovirus infection and disease in Sweden and the relative importance of primary and secondary maternal infections. Scandinavian Journal of Infectious Diseases, 16:129–37, 1984.

64. Stubbs EG. Autistic symptoms in a child with congenital cytomegalovirus infection. Journal of Autism and Childhood Schizophrenia, 8:37–43, 1978.

65. Pavone L, Fiumara A, Bottaro G, Mazzone D, Coleman M. Autism and celiac disease: failure to validate the hypothesis that a link might exist. Biological Psychiatry, 42(1):72–5, 1997.

66. Delong GR, Bean SC, Brown FR. Acquired reversible autistic syndrome in acute encephalopathic illness in children. Archives of Neurology, 38:191–94, 1981.

67. Gillberg C. Do children with autism have March birthdays? Acta Psychiatrica Scandinavica, 82:152–56, 1990.

68. Haymaker W, Pentschew A, Margoles C, Bingham WG. Occurrence of lesions in the temporal lobe in the absence of convulsive seizures. In: Baldwin M, Bailey P, eds. Temporal Lobe Epilepsy. Springfield, IL: C.C. Thomas, pp. 166–202. 1958.

69. Jaeken J, van de Berghe G. An infantile autistic syndrome characterized by the presence of succinylpurines in body fluids. Lancet, 2:1058–61, 1984.

70. McDougle CJ. Effects of tryptophan depletion in drug-free adults with autistic disorder. Archives of General Psychiatry, 53:993–1000, 1996.

71. Plioplys AV et al. Lymphocyst function in autism and Rett syndrome. Neuropsychobiology, 29(1):12–16, 1994.

72. Slikken W Jr., Gaylor DW. Risk assessment strategies for neuroprotective agents. Annals of the New York Academy of Science, 15(765):198–208, 1995.

73. Torrey EF, Hersh SP, McCabe KD. Early childhood psychosis and bleeding

during pregnancy: a prospective study of gravid women and their off-spring. Journal of Autism and Childhood Schizophrenia, 5:287–297, 1975.

74. Rapin I. An 8-year-old boy with autism. Journal of the American Medical Association. 285(13):1749–57, 2001.

75. Lord C, Mulloy C, Wendelboe M, Schopler E. Pre- and perinatal factors in high-functioning females and males with autism. Journal of Autism & Developmental Disorders. 21(2):197–209, 1991.

76. Horvath K, Papadimitriou JC, Rabsztyn A, Drachenberg C, Tildon JT. Gastrointestinal abnormalities in children with autistic disorder. Journal of Pediatrics. 135(5):559–63, 1999.

77. Rapin I. Autistic regression and disintegrative disorder: how important the role of epilepsy? Seminars in Pediatric Neurology. 2(4):278–85, 1995.

78. Rapin I. Autism. New England Journal of Medicine. 337(2):97–104, 1997.

79. Rapin I. An 8-year-old boy with autism. Journal of the American Medical Association. 285(13):1749–57, 2001.

80. Ritvo ER, Freeman BJ, Mason-Brothers A, Mo A, Ritvo AM. Concordance of the syndrome of autism in 40 pairs of afflicted twins. American Journal of Psychiatry, 142:74–77, 1985

81. Bolton P, Rutter M. Genetic influences in autism. International Review of Psychiatry. 2:67–80, 1990.

82. Boss GR, Seegmiller JE. Genetic defects in human purine and pyrimidine metabolism. Annual Review of Genetics, 16:297–328, 1982.

83. Folstein S, Rutter M. Infantile autism: a genetic study of 21 twin pairs. Journal of Child Psychology and Psychiatry. 18:297–321, 1977.

84. Hagerman RJ. Chromosomes, genes, and autism. In: Gillberg C., ed. Diagnosis and Treatment of Autism. New York: Plenum, pp. 105–32, 1989.

85. Nanson JL. Autism in fetal alcohol syndrome: a report of six cases. Alcoholism: Clinical & Experimental Research. 16(3):558–65, 1992.

86. Harris SR, MacKay LL, Osborn JA. Autistic behaviors in offspring of mothers abusing alcohol and other drugs: a series of case reports. Alcoholism: Clinical & Experimental Research. 19(3):660–65, 1995.

87. Aronson M, Hagberg B, Gillberg C. Attention deficits and autistic spectrum problems in children exposed to alcohol during gestation: a follow-up study. Developmental Medicine & Child Neurology. 39(9):583–87, 1997.

88. Stromland K, Nordin V, Miller M, Akerstrom B, Gillberg C. Autism in thalidomide embryopathy: a population study. Developmental Medicine & Child Neurology. 36(4):351–56, 1994.

89. Miller MT, Stromland K, Gillberg C, Johansson M, Nilsson EW. The puzzle of autism: an ophthalmologic contribution. Transactions of the American Ophthalmological Society. 96:369–85, 1998.

90. Rodier PM, Ingram JL, Tisdale B, Croog VJ. Linking etiologies in humans

and animal models: studies of autism. Reproductive Toxicology. 11(2–3): 417–22, 1997.

91. Sever LE. Looking for causes of neural tube defects: where does the environment fit in? Environmental Health Perspectives. 103 Suppl 6:165–71, 1995.

92. Shaw GM, Wasserman CR, O'Malley CD, Nelson V, Jackson RJ. Maternal pesticide exposure from multiple sources and selected congenital anomalies. Epidemiology. 10(1):60–66, 1999.

93. Lynberg MC, Khoury MJ. Interaction between epidemiology and laboratory sciences in the study of birth defects: design of birth defects risk factor surveillance in metropolitan Atlanta. Journal of Toxicology & Environmental Health. 40(2–3):435–44, 1993.

94. Sullivan FM. Impact of the environment on reproduction from conception to parturition. Environmental Health Perspectives. 101 Suppl 2:13–18, 1993.

95. Mastroiacovo P, Mazzone T, Addis A, Elephant E, Carlier P, Vial T, Garbis H, Robert E, Bonati M, Ornoy A, Finardi A, Schaffer C, Caramelli L, Rodriguez-Pinilla E, Clementi M. High vitamin A intake in early pregnancy and major malformations: a multicenter prospective controlled study. Teratology. 59(1):7–11, 1999.

96. Khlood EB, Miyoshi H, Iwata H, Kazusaka A, Kon Y, Hadid AH, Moustafe EK, Ghonim MH, Fujita S. Effects of concurrent exposure to 3-methylcholanthrene and vitamin A on fetal development in rats. Japanese Journal of Veterinary Research. 47(1–2):13–23, 1999.

97. Kitzmiller JL, Gavin LA, Gin GD, Jovanovic-Peterson I, Main EK, Zigrang WD. Preconception care of diabetes: glycemic control prevents congenital anomalies. JAMA. 265:731–36.1991

98. Wiznitzer A, Ayalon N, Hershkovitz R, Khamaisi M, Reece EA, Trischler H, Bashan N. Lipoic acid prevention of neural tube defects in offspring of rats with streptozocin-induced diabetes. American Journal of Obstetrics & Gynecology. 180(1, Pt 1):188–93, 1999.

99. Siman CM, Eriksson UJ. Vitamin E decreases the occurrence of malformations in the offspring of diabetic rats. Diabetes. 46:1054–61. 1997.

100. Wentzel P, Thunberg L, Eriksson UJ. The teratogenic effect of diabetic serum is prevented by supplementation of superoxide dismutase and N-acetylcysteine in rat embryo culture. Diabetologia. 40:7–14. 1997.

101. Baker L, Piddington R, Goldman A, Egler J, Moehing J. Myo-inositol and prostaglandins reverse the glucose inhibition of neural tube fusion in cultured mouse embryos. Diabetologia 33:593–96, 1990.

102. Johnson S. Micronutrient accumulation and depletion in schizophrenia, epilepsy, autism and Parkinson's disease?. Medical Hypotheses. 56(5): 641–45, 2001.

103. Eriksson UJ, Borg LAH. Protection by free oxygen radical-scavenging en-

zymes against glucose-induced embryonic malformations in vitro. Diabetologia. 34:325–31, 1991.

104. Wakefield AJ, Murch SH, Anthony A, Linnell J, et al. Ileal-lymphoid nodular hyperplasia, non-specific colitis, and pervasive developmental disorders in children. Lancet. 351(9103):637–41, 1998.

105. Anonymous. Measles, MMR, and autism: the confusion continues. Lancet. 355(9213):1379, 2000.

106. Anonymous. Lancet. 355(9213):1379, 2000. Ibid.

107. Taylor B, Miller E, Farrington CP, Petropoulos MC, Favot-Mayaud I, Li J, Waight PA. Autism and measles, mumps, and rubella vaccine: no epidemiological evidence for a causal association. Lancet. 353(9169):2026–29, 1999.

108. Fombonne E. Inflammatory bowel disease and autism. Lancet. 351(9107): 955, 1998 Mar 28.

109. Richmond P, Goldblatt D. Autism, inflammatory bowel disease, and MMR vaccine. Lancet. 351(9112):1355–56; discussion 1356, 1998.

110. Vaccines: an issue of trust. Consumer Reports Online. FEAT Daily Newsletter, July 10, 2001.

111. Rimland B. The autism epidemic, vaccinations, and mercury. Journal of Nutritional & Environmental Medicine. 10:261–66, 2000.

112. Bernard S, Enayati A, Redwood L, Roger H, Binstock T. Autism: a novel form of mercury poisoning. ARC Research, July 2000.

113. Vaccines: an issue of trust. Consumer Reports Online. FEAT Daily Newsletter, July 10, 2001.

114. Bernard S, Enayati A, Redwood L, Roger H, Binstock T. Autism: a novel form of mercury poisoning. ARC Research, July 2000.

115. Bernard S, Enayati A, Redwood L, Roger H, Binstock T. Autism: a novel form of mercury poisoning. ARC Research, July 2000.

116. Rimland B. The Autism epidemic, vaccinations, and mercury. Journal of Nutritional & Environmental Medicine. 10:261–66, 2000.

117. Mishnew NJ, Goldstein G, Siegel DJ. Neuropsychologic functioning in autism: profile of a complex information processing disorder. Journal of the International Neuropsychological Society. 3(4):303–16, 1997.

118. Rapin I, Katzman R. Neurobiology of autism. Annals of Neurology. 43(1): 7–14, 1998.

119. Stromland K et al. Developmental Medicine & Child Neurology. 36(4): 351–56, 1994. Op cit.

120. Rodier PM et al. Reproductive Toxicology. 11(2–3):417–22, 1997. Op cit.

121. Rapin I, Katzman R. Neurobiology of autism. Annals of Neurology. 43(1):7–14, 1998.

122. Saugstad LF. A lack of cerebral lateralization in schizophrenia is within the normal variation in brain maturation but indicates late, slow maturation. Schizophrenia Research. 39(3):183–96, 1999.

123. Rapin I. Autism. New England Journal of Medicine. 337(2):97–104, 1997.

124. Rodier PM et al. Reproductive Toxicology. 11(2–3):417–22, 1997. Op cit.

125. Starkstein SE, Vazquez S et al. Blood flow deficits in specific brain areas. Neuropsychiatry Online, 1999.

126. Ohnishi T, Matsuda H, Hashimoto T, Kunihiro T, Nishikawa M, Uema T, Sasaki M. Abnormal regional cerebral blood flow in childhood autism. Brain. 123(Pt 9):1838–44, 2000.

127. O'Banion D, Armstrong B, Cummings RA, Stange J. Disruptive behavior: a dietary approach. Journal of Autism and Childhood Schizophrenia. 8(3):325–37, 1978.

128. Pangborn, JB. Detection and treatment of metabolic dysfunctions related to disordered immune response in autistics; Proceedings of Annual Meeting of National Society for Children and Adults with Autism, San Antonio, Texas. July 8–14, 1984.

129. Pangborn JB. 1984. Ibid.

130. York JL et al. CD4 helper T cell depression in autism. Immunology Letters 25:341–46, 1990.

131. Stubbs EG, Litt M, Lis E, Jackson R, Voth W, Linberg A, Litt R. Adenosine deaminase activity decreased in autism. Journal of the American Academy of Child Psychiatry, 21(1):71–74, 1982.

132. Stubbs EG, Crawford ML, Burger DR, Vanderbrook AA. Depressed lymphocyte responsiveness in autistic children. Journal of Autism and Childhood Schizophrenia. 7:49–55, 1977.

133. Singh VL et al. Antibodies to myelin basic protein in children with autistic behavior. Brain, Behavior, and Immunity, 7(1):97–103, 1993.

134. Singh VK et al. Changes of soluble interleukin-2, interleukin-2 receptor, T8 antigen and interleukin-1 in the serum of autistic children. Clinical Immunology and Immunopathology. 61:448–55, 1991.

135. Warren RP, Foster A, Margaretten NC. Reduced natural killer cell activity in autism. Journal of the American Academy of Child & Adolescent Psychiatry. 26(3):333–35, 1987.

136. Singh VK. Immunotherapy for brain diseases and mental illnesses. Progress in Drug Research. 48:129–46, 1997.

137. Fiumara A, Sciotto A, Barone R, D'Asero G, Munda S, Parano E, Pavone L. Peripheral lymphocyte subsets and other immune aspects in Rett syndrome. Pediatric Neurology, 21(3):619–20, 1999.

138. Park SH, Araki S, Nakata A, Kim YH, Park JA, Tanigawa T, Yokoyama K, Sato H. Effects of occupational metallic mercury vapour exposure on suppressor-inducer (CD4+CD45RA+) T lymphocytes and CD57+CD16+ natural killer cells. International Archives of Occupational & Environmental Health. 73(8):537–42, 2000.

139. Connolly AM, Chez MG, Pestronk A, Arnold ST, Mehta S, Deuel RK.

Serum autoantibodies to brain in Landau-Kleffner variant, autism, and other neurologic disorders. Journal of Pediatrics. 134(5):607–13, 1999.

140. Trottier G, Srivastava L, Walker CD. Etiology of infantile autism: a review of recent advances in genetic and neurobiological research. Journal of Psychiatry and Neuroscience, 24(2):103–15, 1999.

141. Scifo R, Cioni M, Nicolosi A, Batticane N, Tirolo C, Testa N, Quattropani MC, Morale MC, Gallo F, Marchetti B. Opioid-immune interactions in autism: behavioural and immunological assessment during a double-blind treatment with naltrexone. Annali dell Istituto Superiore di Sanita. 32(3): 351–59, 1996.

142. Ryan M. The Advocate: Newsletter of the Autism Society of America, Inc. Sept-Oct. 1995.

143. D'Eufemia P, Celli M, Finocchiaro R, Pacifico L, Viozzi L, Zaccagnini M, Cardi E, Giardini O. Abnormal intestinal permeability in children with autism. Acta Paediatrica. 85(9):1076–79, 1996.

144. Warren RP, Odell JD, Warren WL, Burger RA, Maciulis A, Daniels WW, Torres AR. Brief report: immunoglobulin A deficiency in a subset of autistic subjects. Journal of Autism & Developmental Disorders. 27(2):187–92, 1997.

145. Waring RH. Enzyme and sulfur oxidation deficiencies in autistic children with known food and chemical intolerances. Journal of Orthomolecular Medicine, 8(4), December 1993.

146. Rapin I. Autism. New England Journal of Medicine. 337(2):97–104, 1997.

147. Rapin I. Ibid.

148. Lauritsen M, Mors O, Mortensen PB, Ewald H. Infantile autism and associated autosomal chromosome abnormalities: a register-based study and a literature survey. Journal of Child Psychology and Psychiatry and Allied Disciplines, 40(3):335–45, 1999.

149. Konstantareas MM, Homatidis S. Chromosomal abnormalities in a series of children with autistic disorder. Journal of Autism and Developmental Disorders, 29(4):275–85, 1999.

150. Schroer RJ, Phelan MC, Michaelis RC, Crawford EC, Skinner SA, Cuccaro M, Simensen RJ, Bishop J, Skinner C, Fender D, Stevenson RE. Autism and maternally derived aberrations of chromosome 15q. American Journal of Medical Genetics. 76(4):327–36, 1998.

151. Payton JB, Steele MW, Wenger SL, Minshew NJ. The fragile X marker and autism in perspective. Journal of the American Academy of Child & Adolescent Psychiatry. 28(3):417–21, 1989.

152. Rapin I. An 8-year-old boy with autism. JAMA. 285(13):1749–57, 2001.

153. Hallmayer J, Hebert JM, Spiker D, Lotspeich L, McMahon WM, Petersen PB, Nicholas P, Pingree C, Lin AA, Cavalli-Sforza LL, Risch N,

Ciaranello RD. Autism and the X chromosome. Multipoint sib-pair analysis. Archives of General Psychiatry. 53(11):985–89, 1996.

154. McBride PA, Anderson GM, Shapiro T. Autism research. Bringing together approaches to pull apart the disorder. [letter; comment]. Archives of General Psychiatry. 53(11):980–83, 1996.

155. Trottier G, Srivastava L, Walker CD. Etiology of infantile autism: a review of recent advances in genetic and neurobiological research. Journal of Psychiatry & Neuroscience. 24(2):103–15, 1999.

156. Sanua VD. Infantile autism and childhood schizophrenia: review of the issues from the sociocultural point of view. Social Science & Medicine. 17(21):1633–51, 1983.

157. Healy A. Survey finds autism rate has tripled over six years. FEAT Daily Newsletter, April 23, 2001.

158. Honda H, Shimizu Y, Misumi K, Niimi M, Ohashi Y. Cumulative incidence and prevalence of childhood autism in children in Japan. British Journal of Psychiatry. 169(2):228–35, 1996 Aug. Comment in: British Journal of Psychiatry. 169(5):671–72, 1996.

159. Hurt H, Malmud E, Betancourt LM, Brodsky NL, Giannetta JM. A prospective comparison of developmental outcome of children with in utero cocaine exposure and controls using the Battelle Developmental Inventory. Journal of Developmental & Behavioral Pediatrics. 22(1):27–34, 2001.

160. Duran M, Beemer FA, Van de Heiden C, Korteland J, de Bree PK, Brink M, Wadman SK, Lombeck I. Combined deficiency of xanthine oxidase and sulphite oxidase: a defect of molybdenum metabolism or transport? Journal of Inherited Metabolic Disease. 1(4):175–78, 1978.

161. Wadman SK, Duran M, Beemer FA, Cats BP, Johnson JL, Rajagopalan KV, Saudubray JM, Ogier H, Charpentier C, Berger R et al. Absence of hepatic molybdenum cofactor: an inborn error of metabolism leading to a combined deficiency of sulphite oxidase and xanthine dehydrogenase. Journal of Inherited Metabolic Disease. 6 Suppl 1:78–83, 1983.

162. Van der Heiden C, Beemer FA, Brink W, Wadman SK, Duran M. Simultaneous occurrence of xanthine oxidase and sulfite oxidase deficiency. A molybdenum dependent inborn error of metabolism? Clinical Biochemistry. 12(6):206–8, 1979.

163. Kaplan S, Morris J. Kids at risk. U.S. News & World Report, (online version, 2). June 19, 2000.

164. Edelson SB, Cantor DS. Autism: xenobiotic influences. Journal of Toxicology and Industrial Health. 14(4): 553–63, 1998.

165. Felicetti T. Parents of autistic children: some notes on a chemical connection. Milieu Therapy. 1:13–16, 1981.

166. Niswander KR, Gordon M. The women and their pregnancies. Washing-

ton, DC: U.S. Government Printing Office, (DHEW pub. No. 73–379). 1972.

167. McCann BS. Hemispheric asymmetries and early infantile autism. Journal of Autism and Developmental Disorders, 11:401–11, 1981.

168. Yu ML et al. In utero PCB/PCDF exposure: relation of developmental delay to dysmorphology and dose. Neurotoxicological Teratology, 13:195–202, 1991.

169. Bearer CF. How are children different from adults? Environmental Health Perspectives. 103 Suppl 6:7–12, 1995.

170. Aaronson M, Hagberg B, Gillberg C. Attention deficits and autistic spectrum problems in children exposed to alcohol during gestation: a follow-up study. Developmental Medicine & Child Neurology. 39(9):583–87, 1997.

171. Baron-Cohen S, Allen J, Gillberg C. Can autism be detected at 18 months? The needle, the haystack, and the CHAT. British Journal of Pyschiatry. 161:839–43, 1992.

Chapter 4

1. Colborn T, Dumanoski D, Myers JP. Our stolen future. New York: Plume/Penguin Books, 1997.

2. Lappe M. Toxicological perspectives. In: Chemical Deception. San Francisco: Sierra Club Books, p. 6, 1991.

3. National Institute of Environmental Health Sciences. Environment and disease: medicine for the layman. NIEHS Pamphlet: Chemicals and Human Disease. 2001.

4. Claudio L. NIEHS investigates links between children, the environment, and neurotoxicity. Environmental Health Perspectives. 109(6):258–61, 2001.

5. Claudio L. Environmental Health Perspectives. 2001. Ibid.

6. Lemasters GK, Perreault SD, Hales BF, Hatch M, Hirshfield AN, Hughes CL, Kimmel GL, Lamb JC, Pryor JL, Rubin C, Seed JG. Workshop to identify critical windows of exposure for children's health: reproductive health in children and adolescents work group summary. Environmental Health Perspectives. 108 Suppl 3:505–9, 2000.

7. Commission on Life Sciences, National Academy of Sciences. Toxicity testing: strategies to determine needs and priorities. National Academy Press, Washington DC. 1984.

8. Claudio L, Bearer CF, Walinga D. Assessment of the U.S. Environmental Protection Agency methods for identification of hazards to developing organisms, part II: the developmental toxicity testing guideline. American Journal of Internal Medicine. 35:554–63, 1999.

9. Lappe M. Toxicological perspectives, p. 7, 1991. Op cit.

10. Claudio L. Environmental Health Perspectives. 2001. Op cit.

11. DiGiulio R. Duke University Medical Center, press release. 1999.

12. Center for Children's Health and the Environment, Mount Sinai School of Medicine. Children's vulnerability to toxins in the environment. 2001.

13. World Resources Institute, UNEP, UNDP, World Bank. World resources 1998–1999. Environmental change and human health. New York: Oxford University Press. 1998.

14. Goldman LK, Koduru S. Chemicals in the environment and developmental toxicity to children: a public health and policy perspective. Environmental Health Perspectives. 108 Suppl 3:443–48, 2000.

15. National Research Council. Pesticides in the diets of infants and children. Washington: National Academy Press, 1993.

16. Center for Children's Health and the Environment. Ibid. 2001.

17. Gardella C. Lead exposure in pregnancy: a review of the literature and argument for routine prenatal screening. Obstetrical & Gynecological Survey. 56(4):231–38, 2001.

18. Weiss B, Landrigan PJ. The Developing brain and the environment. Environmental Health Perspectives Supplement, 108(3):373–74, 2000.

19. Jacobsen JL, Jacobsen SW. Intellectual impairment and children exposed to polychorinated biphenyls in utero. New England Journal of Medicine. 335:783–89, 1996.

20. Clarkson TW. The toxicology of mercury. Critical Reviews in Clinical Laboratory Sciences. 34(4):369–403, 1997.

21. Myers GJ, Davidson PW. Prenatal methylmercury exposure and children: neurologic, developmental, and behavioral research. Environmental Health Perspectives. 106 Suppl 3:841–47, 1998.

22. Myers GJ, Davidson PW. Does methylmercury have a role in causing developmental disabilities in children? Environmental Health Perspectives. 108 Suppl 3:413–20, 2000.

23. Children and the polluted environment. Report for Center for Children's Health and the Environment, Department of Community and Preventive Medicine, Mount Sinai School of Medicine, New York. (childenvironment.org) 2001.

24. NIEHS working group. A research-oriented framework for risk assessment and prevention of children's exposure to environmental toxicants. Environmental Health Perspectives. 107(6):510, 1999.

25. Rice D, Barone S. Critical periods of vulnerability for the developing nervous system: evidence from humans and animal models. Environmental Health Perspectives. 108 Suppl 3:511–33, 2000.

26. Colborn T, Dumanoski D, Myers JP. Our Stolen Future. New York: Plume/Penguin Books, p. 106, 1997.

27. Steinman D, Wisner RM. Living Healthy in a Toxic World. NY, NY: The Berkeley Publishing Group. 1996.

28. Steinman D, Wisner RM. Living Healthy in a Toxic World. NY, NY: The Berkeley Publishing Group. 1996.

29. Anderson JH. Reactions to carpet emissions: a case series. Journal of Nutritional & Environmental Medicine. 7:177–85, 1997.

30. Kilburn KH, Warshaw RH. Prevalence of symptoms of systemic lupus erythematosus (SLE) and of fluorescent antinuclear antibodies associated with chronic exposure to trichloroethylene and other chemicals in well water. Environmental Research. 57:1–9, 1992.

31. Landtblom AM, Flodin U, Soderfeldt B, Wolfson C, Axelson O. Organic solvents and multiple sclerosis: a synthesis of the current evidence. Epidemiology. 7(4):429–33, 1996.

32. Windham, B. Effects of toxic metals on learning ability and behavior. CQS Health Alert & Toxic Alert. URL: www.cqs.com/toxicmetals.htm. 2002.

33. Windham B. Annotated bibliography of exposure and health effects from amalgam fillings. URL: www.positivehealth.com/permit/Articles/Dentist/wind45.htm. 1997.

34. Windham B. Effects of toxic metals on learning ability and behavior. CQS Health Alert & Toxic Alert. URL: www.cqs.com/toxicmetals.htm. 2002.

35. Windham B. Effects of toxic metals on learning ability and behavior. CQS Health Alert & Toxic Alert. URL: www.cqs.com/toxicmetals.htm. 2002.

36. Goyer RA. National Institute of Environmental Health Sciences. Toxic and essential metal interactions. Annual Review of Nutrition. 17:37–50 1997. Nutrition and metal toxicity. American Journal of Clinical Nutrition. 61 (Suppl 3):646S–50S, 1995.

37. Weiner JA, Nylander M. Aspect on health risks of mercury from dental amalgams. Chapter 30, 469–86 in Toxicology of Metals, ed. Louis W. Chang, Laszlo Magos, Tsuguyoshi Suzuki.

38. Windham B. Annotated bibliography: health effects related to mercury from amalgam fillings and documented clinical results of replacement of amalgam fillings. 1999.

39. Sanfeliu C, Sebastia J, Kim SU. Methylmercury neurotoxicity in cultures of human neurons, astrocytes, neuroblastoma cells. NeuroToxicology. 22: 317–27, 2001.

40. Myers GJ, Davidson PW, Cox C, Shamlaye C, Cernichiari E, Clarkson TW. Twenty-seven years studying the human neurotoxicity of methylmercury exposure. Environmental Research. 83(3):275–85, 2000.

41. Myers GJ, Davidson PW. Does methylmercury have a role in causing developmental disabilities in children? Environmental Health Perspectives. 108 Suppl 3:413–20, 2000.

42. Menkes DB, Fawcett JP. So easily lead? Health effects of gasoline additives. Environmental Health Perspectives, 105(3):270–72, 1997.

43. Accardo P, Whitman B, Jefferies C, Rolfe U. Autism and plumbism: a possible association. Clinical Pediatrics, 27(1):41–44, January 1988.

44. Needleman HL, Schell A, Bellinger D, Leviton A, Allred EN. The long-term effects of exposure to low doses of lead in childhood. An 11-year follow-up report. New England Journal of Medicine. 322:83–88, 1990.

45. Silva PA, Hughes P, Williams S, Faed JM. Blood lead, intelligence, reading attainment, and behaviour in eleven-year-old children in Dunedin, New Zealand. Journal of Child Psychology and Psychiatry. 29:43–52, 1988.

46. Centers for Disease Control and Prevention. Update: blood lead levels—United States, 1991–1994. MMWR. 46(07):141–46, 1997.

47. Schwartz J. Low-level lead exposure and children's IQ: a meta-analysis and search for a threshold. Environmental Research. 65:42–55, 1994.

48. Raloff J. Even low lead in kids has a high IQ cost. Science News. 159:277.

49. Wasserman GA, Liu X, Lolacono NJ, Factor-Litvak P, Kline JK, Popovac D, Morina N, Musabegovic A, Vrenezi N, Capuni-Paracka S, Lekic V, Preteni-Redjepi E, Hadzialjevic S, Slavkovich V, Graziano JH. Lead exposure and intelligence in seven-year-old children: the Yugoslavia prospective study. Environmental Health Perspectives, 105(9):956–62, 1997.

50. Needleman HL et al. Bone lead levels and delinquent behavior. Journal of the American Medical Association. 275(5):363–69, 1996.

51. Gardella C. Lead exposure in pregnancy: a review of the literature and argument for routine prenatal screening. Obstetrical & Gynecological Survey. 56(4):231–38, 2001.

52. Crinnion WJ. Environmental medicine, part 1: The human burden of environmental toxins and their common health effects. Alternative Medicine Reviews. 5(1):52–63, 2000.

53. Spencer PS, Schaumburg HH. Organic solvent neurotoxicity: facts and research needs. Scandinavian Journal of Work, Environment & Health. 11 Suppl 1:53–60, 1985.

54. Baelum J. Human solvent exposure: factors influencing the pharmacokinetics and acute toxicity. Pharmacology & Toxicology. 68 Suppl 1:1–36, 1991.

55. Osterberg K, Orbaek P, Karlson B, Seger L, Akesson B, Bergendorf U. Psychological test performance during experimental challenge to toluene and n-butyl acetate in cases of solvent-induced toxic encephalopathy. Scandinavian Journal of Work, Environment & Health. 26(3):219–26, 2000.

56. Colvin M, Myers J, Nell V, Rees D, Cronje R. A cross-sectional survey of neurobehavioral effects of chronic solvent exposure on workers in a paint manufacturing plant. Environmental Research. 63(1):122–32, 1993.

57.   Triebig G. Occupational neurotoxicology of organic solvents and solvent mixtures. Neurotoxicology & Teratology. 11(6):575–78, 1989.

58.   Kraut A, Lilis R, Marcus M, Valciukas JA, Wolff MS, Landrigan PJ. Neurotoxic effects of solvent exposure on sewage treatment workers. Archives of Environmental Health. 43(4):263–68, 1988.

59.   Triebig G, Barocka A, Erbguth F, Holl R, Lang C, Lehrl S, Rechlin T, Weidenhammer W, Weltle D. Neurotoxicity of solvent mixtures in spray painters. II. Neurologic, psychiatric, psychological, and neuroradiologic findings. International Archives of Occupational & Environmental Health. 64(5):361–72, 1992.

60.   Daniell W, Stebbins A, O'Donnell J, Horstman SW, Rosenstock L. Neuropsychological performance and solvent exposure among car body repair shop workers. British Journal of Industrial Medicine. 50(4):368–77, 1993.

61.   Arlien-Soborg P. Solvent Neurotoxicity. Chapter 5, N-hexane, 155–83. CRC Press.

62.   Gralewicz S, Wiaderna D. Behavioral effects following subacute inhalation exposure to m-xylene or trimethylbenzene in the rat: a comparative study. NeuroToxicology. 22:79–89, 2001.

63.   Raloff J. Picturing pesticides' impacts on kids. Science News, vol. 153, June 6, 1998, 358. Reporting on study published in June 1998 issue of Environmental Health Perspectives, June 1998.

64.   Montague P. Pesticides and aggression. Our Toxic Times, vol. 10, no. 6, issue 108, 1-5, June 1999. Reporting on study: Porter WP, Jaeger JW, Carlson IH. Endocrine, immune and behavioral effects of aldicarb (carbamate), atrazine (triazine) and nitrate (fertilizer) mixtures at groundwater concentrations. Toxicology and Industrial Health 15(1 & 2):133–50, 1999.

65.   Bearer CF. The special and unique vulnerability of children to environmental hazards. NeuroToxicology 21(6):925–34, 2000.

66.   Bearer CF. The special and unique vulnerability of children to environmental hazards. NeuroToxicology 21(6):925–34, 2000.

67.   Fact Sheet: Handle with Care: Children and Environmental Carcinogens. Natural Resources Defense Council.

68.   Bearer CF. The special and unique vulnerability of children to environmental hazards. NeuroToxicology 21(6):925–34, 2000.

69.   Fact Sheet: Handle with care: children and environmental carcinogens. Natural Resources Defense Council.

70.   Bearer CF. The special and unique vulnerability of children to environmental hazards. NeuroToxicology 21(6):925–34, 2000.

71.   Bearer CF. The special and unique vulnerability of children to environmental hazards. NeuroToxicology 21(6):925–34, 2000.

72.   Bearer CF. The special and unique vulnerability of children to environmental hazards. NeuroToxicology 21(6):925–34, 2000.

73. Jacobsen JL, Jacobsen SW. New England Journal of Medicine. 335: 783–89, 1996. Op cit.

74. Colborn T, Dumanoski D, Myers, JP. Our stolen future. New York: Plume/ Penguin Books, pp. 251–52, 1997.

75. Colborn T, Dumanoski D, Myers, JP. Our stolen future. New York: Plume/ Penguin Books, p. 251, 1997.

76. National Institute of Environmental Health Sciences. Kids 'n' the environmental health sciences: NIEHS Fact Sheet #5: Finding ways to help a "vulnerable population." February 1997.

77. Goldman LR. Linking research and policy to ensure children's environmental health. Environmental Health Perspectives. 106 (Supplement 3): 857–62. 1998.

78. Center for Children's Health and the Environment, Mount Sinai School of Medicine. Endocrine Disruptors and Children's Health. 2001.

79. Ashford NA, Miller CS. Chemical exposures: low levels and high stakes. New York: John Wiley, 1998.

80. Ashford NA, Miller CS. Chemical exposures: low levels and high stakes. New York: John Wiley, 1998.

81. Betz Al. An overview of the multiple functions of the blood-brain barrier. NIDA Research Monograph. 120:54–72, 1992.

Chapter 5

1. Pfeiffer SI, Norton J, Nelson L, Shott S. Efficacy of vitamin B_6 and magnesium in the treatment of autism: a methodology review and summary of outcomes. Journal of Autism & Developmental Disorders. 25(5):481–93, 1995.

2. Wilkinson J Clapper ML. Detoxication enzymes and chemoprevention. Proceedings of the Society for Experimental Biology & Medicine. 216(2):192–200, 1997.

3. Martin WJ. Stealth viruses as neuropathogens. College of American Pathologists.

4. Warren RP, Foster A, Margaretten NC. Reduced natural killer cell activity in autism. Journal of the American Academy of Child & Adolescent Psychiatry. 26(3):333–5, 1987.

5. van Gent T, Heijnen CJ, Treffers PD. Autism and the immune system. Journal of Child Psychology & Psychiatry & Allied Disciplines. 38(3): 337–49, 1997.

6. Comi AM, Zimmerman AW, Frye VH, Law PA, Peeden JN. Familial clustering of autoimmune disorders and evaluation of medical risk factors in autism. Journal of Child Neurology. 14(6):388–94, 1999.

7. Benady S. Experts redefine autism as a systemic illness. Feat Daily Newsletter, July 28, 2001.

8. Todd RD, Hickok JM, Anderson GM, Cohen DJ. Antibrain antibodies in infantile autism. Biological Psychiatry. 23:644–47, 1988.

9. Singh VK, Warren R, Averett R, Ghaziuddin M. Circulating autoantibodies to neuronal and glial filament proteins in autism. Pediatric Neurology. 17(1):88–90, 1997.

10. Connolly AM, Chez MG, Pestronk A, Arnold ST, Mehta S, Deuel RK. Serum autoantibodies to brain in Landau-Kleffner variant, autism, and other neurologic disorders. Journal of Pediatrics. 134(5):607–13, 1999.

11. Nevsimalova S, Tauberova A, Doutlik S, Kucera V, Dlouha O. A role of autoimmunity in the etiopathogenesis of Landau-Kleffner Syndrome? Brain & Development, 14(5):342–45, 1992.

12. Sakic B, Szechtman H, Denburg JA. Neurobehavioral alterations in autoimmune mice. Neuroscience & Biobehavioral Reviews. 21(3):327–40, 1997.

13. Hornig M, Lipkin WI. Infectious and immune factors in the pathogenesis of neurodevelopmental disorders: epidemiology, hypotheses, and animal models. Mental Retardation & Developmental Disabilities Research Reviews. 7(3):200–10, 2001.

14. Benady S. Experts redefine autism as a systemic illness. Feat Daily Newsletter, July 28, 2001.

15. Gupta S, Aggarwal S, Rashanravan B, Lee T. Th1- and Th2-like cytokines in CD4+ and CD8+ T cells in autism. Journal of Neuroimmunology 85(1):106–9, 1998.

16. Kroemer G, Hirsch F, Gonzalez-Garcia A, Martinez C. Differential involvement of Th1 and Th2 cytokines in autoimmune diseases. Autoimmunity. 24(1):25–33, 1996.

17. Heo Y, Lee WT, Lawrence DA. In vivo the environmental pollutants lead and mercury induce oligoclonal T cell responses skewed toward type-2 reactivities. Cellular Immunology. 179(2):185–95, 1997.

18. Hu H, Moller G, Abedi-Valugerdi M. Mechanism of mercury-induced autoimmunity: both T helper 1- and T helper 2-type responses are involved. Immunology. 96(3):348–57, 1999.

19. Pollard KM, Pearson DL, Hultman P, Deane TN, Lindh U, Kono DH. Xenobiotic acceleration of idiopathic systemic autoimmunity in lupus-prone bxsb mice. Environmental Health Perspectives. 109(1):27–33, 2001.

20. Warren RP, Yonk LJ, Burger RA, Cole P, Odell JD, Warren WL, White E, Singh VK. Deficiency of suppressor-inducer (CD4+CD45RA+) T cells in autism. Immunological Investigations. 19(3): 245–51, 1990.

21. Griffin JM, Blossom SJ, Jackson SK, Gilbert KM, Pumford NR. Trichloroethylene accelerates an autoimmune response by Th1T cell activation in MRL+/+ mice. Immunopharmacology. 46:123–37, 2000.

22. Plioplys AV. Intravenous immunoglobulin treatment of autism. Journal of Child Neurology. 13(2): 79–82, February 199ᴕ with

23. Boddaert N, Zilbovicius M, Belin P, Thivard L, Poline JB, Ribeiro ᴵ. Barthelemy C, Samson Y. Temporal lobe dysfunction in autism: a pet auditory activation study. Abstract in FEAT Daily Newsletter, Nov. 15, 2000.

24. Connolly AM, Chez MG, Pestronk A, Arnold ST, Mehta S, Deuel RK. Serum autoantibodies to brain in Landau-Kleffner variant, autism, and other neurologic disorders. Journal of Pediatrics. 134(5):607–13, 1999.

25. Baron J, Voigt JM, Whitter TB, Kawabata TT, Knapp SA, Guengerich FP, Jakoby WB. Identification of intratissue sites for xenobiotic activation and detoxication. Advances in Experimental Medicine & Biology. 197:119–44, 1986.

26. Raiten DJ, Massaro T. Perspectives on the nutritional ecology of autistic children. Journal of Autism & Developmental Disorders. 16(2):133–43, 1986.

27. Mercer ME, Holder MD. Food cravings, endogenous opioid peptides, and food intake: a review. Appetite. 29(3):325–52, 1997.

28. Sher L. Autistic disorder and the endogenous opioid system. Medical Hypotheses. 48(5):413–4, 1997.

29. Scifo R, Cioni M, Nicolosi A, Batticane N, Tirolo C, Testa N, Quattropani MC, Morale MC, Gallo F, Marchetti B. Opioid-immune interactions in autism: behavioural and immunological assessment during a double-blind treatment with naltrexone. Annali dell Istituto Superiore di Sanita. 32(3): 351–59, 1996.

30. O'Banion D, Armstrong B, Cummings RA, Stange J. Disruptive behavior: a dietary approach. Journal of Autism & Childhood Schizophrenia. 8(3): 325–37, 1978.

31. Worth J. Autism: is it an allergic disease? Conference of the Allergy Research Foundation, London, Nov. 18, 1999. Journal of Nutritional & Environmental Medicine. 10:321–24, 2000.

32. Dolske MC, Spollen J, McKay S, Lancashire E, Tolbert L. A preliminary trial of ascorbic acid as supplemental therapy for autism. Progress in Neuro-Psychopharmacology & Biological Psychiatry. 17(5):765–74, September 1993.

33. Pfeiffer SI, Norton J, Nelson L, Shott S. Efficacy of vitamin B_6 and magnesium in the treatment of autism: a methodology review and summary of outcomes. Journal of Autism & Developmental Disorders. 25(5):481–93, 1995.

34. LaPerchia P. Behavioral disorders, learning disabilities and megavitamin therapy. Adolescence. 22(87):729–38, 1987.

35. Martineau J, Barthelemy C, Garreau B, Lelord G. Vitamin B_6, magnesium,

B_6-Mg: therapeutic effects in childhood autism. Biological and atry. 20(5):467–78, 1985.

Moreno-Fuenmayor H, Borjas L, Arrieta A, Valera V, Socorro-Candanoza L. Plasma excitatory amino acids in autism. Investigacion Clinica. 37(2): 113–28, June 1996.

37. Raiten DJ et al. Vitamin and trace element assessment of autistic and learning disabled children. Nutrition and Behavior. 2:9, 1984.

38. Schauss A. Nutrition and Behavior. New Canaan, CT: Keats Publishing, Inc., p. 19. 1985.

39. Frager J et al. A double-blind study of vitamin B_6 in Down's sydrome infants, part 2: cortical auditory evoked potentials. Journal of Mental Deficiency Research. 29:241, 1985.

40. Schauss A. 1985. Op cit., p. 22.

41. Johnson S. Micronutrient accumulation and depletion in schizophrenia, epilepsy, autism and Parkinson's disease? Medical Hypotheses. 56(5): 641–45, 2001.

42. Shrestha KP, Carrera AE. Hair trace elements and mental retardation among children. Archives of Environmental Health. 43(6):396. 1988.

43. Klevay L et al. Evidence of dietary copper and zinc deficiencies. Journal of the American Medical Association. 241:1916. 1979.

44. Dreosti IE, Smith RM (eds). Neurobiology of the Trace Elements (Vol. I and II). Clifton, N.J.: The Humana Press, 1983.

45. Pfeiffer CC. Mental and Elemental Nutrients. New Canaan, Conn.: Keats Publishing Co. 1975.

46. Chandra RK. Trace Elements in Nutrition of Children. New York: Raven Press. 1985.

47. D'Eufemia P, Celli M, Finocchiaro R, Pacifico L, Viozzi L, Zaccagnini M, Cardi E, Giardini O. Abnormal intestinal permeability in children with autism. Acta Paediatrica. 85(9):1076–9, 1996.

48. Waring RH. Enzyme and sulfur oxidation deficiencies in autistic children with known food and chemical intolerances. Journal of Orthomolecular Medicine. 8(4), December1993.

49. Bland JS, Bralley JA. Nutritional upregulation of hepatic detoxication enzymes. Journal of Applied Nutrition. 44(3&4), 1992.

50. Talalay P, Prochaska HJ, Spencer SR. Regulation of enzymes that detoxify the electrophilic forms of chemical carcinogens. Princess Takamatsu Symposia. 21:177–87, 1990.

51. Prochaska HJ, Santamaria AB, Talalay P. Rapid detection of inducers of enzymes that protect against carcinogens. Proceedings of the National Academy of Sciences of the United States of America. 89(6):2394–8, 1992.

52. McFadden SA. Phenotypic variation in xenobiotic metabolism and adverse

environmental response: focus on sulfur-dependent detoxication pathways. Toxicology. 111(1–3):43–65, 1996.

53. Worth J. Autism: is it an allergic disease? Conference of the allergy research foundation, London, November 18, 1999. Journal of Nutritional & Environmental Medicine. 10:321–24, 2000.

54. Worth J. Autism: is it an allergic disease? Conference of the allergy research foundation, London, November 18, 1999. Journal of Nutritional & Environmental Medicine. 10:321–24, 2000.

55. Bernard S, Enayati A, Redwood L, Roger H, Binstock T. Autism: a novel form of mercury poisoning. ARC Research. 2000.

56. Accardo P, Whitman B, Caul J, Rolfe U. Autism and plubmism: a possible association. Clinical Pediatrics. 27(1):41–44, January 1988.

57. Marlowe M, Errera J, Jacobs J. Increased lead and cadmium burdens among mentally retarded children and children with borderline intelligence. American Journal of Mental Deficiency. 87(5):477–83, March 1983; & Journal of Special Education. 16:87–99, 1982.

58. Gardella C. Lead exposure in pregnancy: a review of the literature and argument for routine prenatal screening. Obstetrical & Gynecological Survey. 56(4):231–8, 2001.

59. Annau Z, Cuomo V. Mechanisms of neurotoxicity and their relationship to behavioral changes. Toxicology. 49(2–3):219–25, 1988.

Chapter 6

1. Sobarzo C, Bustos-Obregon E. Sperm quality in mice acutely treated with parathion. Asian Journal of Andrology. 2(2):147–50, 2000.

2. Shi Q, Ko E, Barclay L, Hoang T, Rademaker A, Martin R. Cigarette smoking and aneuploidy in human sperm. Molecular Reproduction & Development. 59(4):417–21, 2001.

3. Jarow JP, Detection of oxidative DNA damage in human sperm and the association with cigarette smoking. Journal of Urology. 159(5):1774–75, 1998.

4. Dawson EB, Ritter S, Harris WA, Evans DR, Powell LC. Comparison of sperm viability with seminal plasma metal levels. Biological Trace Element Research. 64(1–3):215–19, 1998.

5. Mohamed MK, Lee WI, Mottet NK, Burbacher TM. Laser light-scattering study of the toxic effects of methylmercury on sperm motility. Journal of Andrology. 7(1):11–15, 1986.

6. Ackerman DJ, Reinecke AJ, Els HJ, Grobler DG, Reinecke SA. Sperm abnormalities associated with high copper levels in impala (Aepyceros melampus). Ecotoxicology & Environmental Safety. 43(3):261–16, 1999.

7. Sokol RZ, Okuda H, Nagler HM, Berman N. Lead exposure in vivo alters

the fertility potential of sperm in vitro. Toxicology & Applied Pharmacology. 124(2):310–16, 1994.

8. Assennato G, Paci C, Baser ME, Molinini R, Candela RG, Altamura BM, Giorgino R. Sperm count suppression without endocrine dysfunction in lead-exposed men. Archives of Environmental Health. 42(2):124–27, 1987.

9. Fredricsson B, Moller L, Pousette A, Westerholm R. Human sperm motility is affected by plasticizers and diesel particle extracts. Pharmacology & Toxicology. 72(2):128–33, 1993.

10. Drife JO. The effects of drugs on sperm. Drugs. 33(6):610–22, 1987.

11. Washington WJ, Murthy RC, Doye A, Eugene K, Brown D, Bradley I. Induction of morphologically abnormal sperm in rats exposed to O-Xylene. Archives of Andrology. 11(3):233–37, 1983.

12. de Lamirande E, Gagnon C. Reactive oxygen species and human spermatozoa. I. Effects on the motility of intact spermatozoa and on sperm axonemes. Journal of Andrology. 13(5):368–78, 1992.

13. Siegel I, Dudkiewicz AB, Friberg J, Suarez M, Gleicher N. Inhibition of sperm motility and agglutination of sperm cells by free fatty acids in whole semen. Fertility & Sterility. 45(2):273–79, 1986.

14. Zenzes MT. Smoking and reproduction: gene damage to human gametes and embryos. Human Reproduction Update. 6(2):122–31, 2000.

15. Makler A, Reiss J, Stoller J, Blumenfeld Z, Brandes JM. Use of a sealed minichamber for direct observation and evaluation of the in vitro effect of cigarette smoke on sperm motility. Fertility & Sterility. 59(3):645–51, 1993.

16. Englert Y. [Influence of environmental factors on fertility: example of the diminution of sperm quality]. [French] Revue Medicale de Bruxelles. 19(4):A372–73, 1998.

17. Jarrell JF, McMahon A, Villeneuve D, Franklin C, Singh A, Valli VE, Bartlett S. Hexachlorobenzene toxicity in the monkey primordial germ cell without induced porphyria. Reproductive Toxicology. 7(1):41–47, 1993.

18. Kimmel CA, Makris SL. Recent developments in regulatory requirements for developmental toxicology. Toxicology Letters. 120(1–3):73–82, 2001.

19. Bearer CF. The special and unique vulnerability of children to environmental hazards. NeuroToxicology 21(6):925–34, 2000.

20. Gillberg C, Coleman M. Chapter 19, The neurology of autism, in The Biology of the Autistic Syndromes, 3rd ed. Clinics in Developmental Medicine 153(4). London: Mac Keith Press, pp. 302–4, 2000.

21. Ibid.

22. Ibid.

23. Ibid.

24. Gillberg C, Coleman M. Op cit.

25. Bearer CF. The special and unique vulnerability of children to environmental hazards. NeuroToxicology. 21(6):925–34, 2000.

26. Hans SL. Prenatal drug exposure: behavioral functioning in late childhood and adolescence. NIDA Research Monograph. 164:261–76, 1996.

27. Lewis M, Worobey J, Ramsay DS, McCormack MK. Prenatal exposure to heavy metals: effect on childhood cognitive skills and health status. Pediatrics. 89(6, Pt 1):1010–15, 1992.

28. Goyer RA. Results of lead research: prenatal exposure and neurological consequences. Environmental Health Perspectives. 104(10):1050–54, 1996.

29. Bearer CF. The special and unique vulnerability of children to environmental hazards. NeuroToxicology. 21(6):925–34, 2000.

30. Harris SR, MacKay LL, Osborn JA. Autistic behaviors in offspring of mothers abusing alcohol and other drugs: a series of case reports. Alcoholism: Clinical & Experimental Research. 19(3):660–65, 1995.

31. Gillberg C, Coleman M. Chapter 11, Double syndromes, in The biology of the autistic syndromes, 3rd ed. Clinics in Developmental Medicine. 153(4). London: Mac Keith Press, pp. 166–67, 2000.

32. Stromland K, Nordin V, Miller M, Akerstrom B, Gillberg C. Autism in thalidomide embryopathy: a population study. Developmental Medicine & Child Neurology. 36(4):351–56, 1994.

33. Rodier PM, Ingram JL, Tisdale B, Croog VJ. Linking etiologies in humans and animal models: studies of autism. Reproductive Toxicology. 11(2–3):417–22, 1997.

34. Nanson JL. Autism in fetal alcohol syndrome: a report of six cases. Alcoholism: Clinical & Experimental Research. 16(3):558–65, 1992.

35. Aronson M, Hagberg B, Gillberg C. Attention deficits and autistic spectrum problems in children exposed to alcohol during gestation: a follow-up study. Developmental Medicine & Child Neurology. 39(9):583–87, 1997.

36. Ammenheuser MM, Berenson AB, Babiak AE, Singleton CR, Whorton EB Jr. Frequencies of hprt mutant lymphocytes in marijuana-smoking mothers and their newborns. Mutation Research. 403(1–2):55–64, 1998.

37. Sasco AJ, Vainio H. From in utero and childhood exposure to parental smoking to childhood cancer: a possible link and the need for action. Human & Experimental Toxicology. 18(4):192–201, 1999.

38. Bearer CF. The special and unique vulnerability of children to environmental hazards. NeuroToxicology. 21(6):925–34, 2000.

39. Marselos M, Tomatis L. Diethylstilboestrol: II, pharmacology, toxicology and carcinogenicity in experimental animals. European Journal of Cancer. 29A(1):149–55, 1992.

40. McKee RH, Pasternak SJ, Traul KA. Developmental toxicity of EDS recycle solvent and fuel oil. Toxicology. 46(2):205–15, 1987.

41. Brown DW. Autism, Asperger's syndrome and the Crick-Mitchison theory of the biological function of REM sleep. Medical Hypotheses. 47(5):399–403, 1996.

42. Schantz SL. Developmental neurotoxicity of PCBs in humans: what do we know and where do we go from here? Neurotoxicology & Teratology. 18(3):217–27; discussion 229–76, 1996.

43. Kholkute SD, Rodriguez J, Dukelow WR. Reproductive toxicity of Aroclor-1254: effects on oocyte, spermatozoa, in vitro fertilization, and embryo development in the mouse. Reproductive Toxicology. 8(6):487– 93, 1994.

44. Gladen BC, Ragan NB, Rogan WJ. Pubertal growth and development and prenatal and lactational exposure to polychlorinated biphenyls and dichloro-diphenyl dichloroethene. Journal of Pediatrics. 136(4):490–96, 2000.

45. Riggs BS, Bronstein AC, Kulig K, Archer PG, Rumack BH. Acute acetaminophen overdose during pregnancy. Obstetrics Gynecology. 74:247–53, 1989.

46. King JC. Physiology of pregnancy and nutrient metabolism. American Journal of Clinical Nutrition. 71(suppl):1218S–25S, 2000.

47. King JC, Sachet P. Preface to "Pregnancy and Nutrition" issue. American Journal of Clinical Nutrition. 71(suppl):1217S, 2000.

48. Scholl TO, Johnson WG. Folic acid: influence on the outcome of pregnancy. American Journal of Clinical Nutrition. 71(suppl):1295S–303S, 2000.

49. Public Health Assessment, Brick Township Investigation (a/k/a Brick Township Autism Investigation. Superfund Site Assessment Branch, Division of Health Assessment and Consultation, Agency for Toxic Substances and Disease Registry. 2000.

50. King JC, P Sachet. Op. cit.

51. Bailey LB. New standard for dietary folate intake in pregnant women. American Journal of Clinical Nutrition. 71(suppl):1304S–7S, 2000.

52. King JC. 2000. Op. cit.

Chapter 7

1. Schaumburg HH, Spencer PS. Recognizing neurotoxic disease. Neurology. 37:276–78, 1987.

2. Ibid.

Chapter 8

1. Connors CK. Feeding the brain: how foods affect children. New York: Plenum Press, p. 3, 1989.

2. Fernstrom JD. How food affects your brain. Nutrition Action Newsletter. Center for Science in the Public Interest, December 1979.

3. U.S. Senate Select Committee on Nutrition and Human Needs. Nutrition and mental health. Berkeley, CA: Parker House, 1980.

4. Raifman M. Director, Pediatrics at Peninsula Hospital Center, Far Rockaway, N.Y., Plenary Address to the American Public Health Association. Cited by R. Mendelsohn in How to Raise a Healthy Child in Spite of Your Doctor. Chicago: Contemporary Books, Inc, p. 56, 1984.

5. Benton D, Roberts G. Effect of vitamin and mineral supplementation on intelligence of a sample of schoolchildren. Lancet 1(8578): 140–43, 1988.

6. Sankar DVS. Plasma levels of folates, riboflavin, vitamin B_6 and ascorbate in severely disturbed children. Journal of Autism and Developmental Disorders, 9:73–82, 1979.

7. Rimland B. An orthomolecular study of psychotic children. Journal of Orthomolecular Psychiatry, 3: 3371–77, 1974.

8. Rimland B, Callaway E, Dreyfus P. The effects of high doses of vitamin B_6 on autistic children: a double-blind crossover study. American Journal of Psychiatry, 135: 472–75, 1978.

9. Gillberg C, Coleman M. The biology of the autistic syndromes. Clinics in Developmental Medicine No. 153 (4). London: Mac Keith Press, p. 279, 2000.

10. Balch JF, Balch PA. Prescription for nutritional healing: A-to-Z guide to supplements. New York: Avery Publishing Group, p. 95, 1998.

11. Murray MT. Encyclopedia of nutritional supplements. Rocklin, CA: Prima Publishing, p. 139, 1996.

12. Murray, p. 365. Ibid.

13. Murray, p. 291. Ibid.

14. Fukuda K, Ohta T. Yamazoe Y. Grapefruit component interacting with rat and human P450 CYP3A: possible involvement of non-flavonoid components in drug interaction. Biological & Pharmaceutical Bulletin. 1997; 20(5):560–64.

Afterword

1. Claudio L. NIEHS investigates links between children, the environment, and neurotoxicity. Environmental Health Perspectives. 109(6):258–61, 2001

2. Goldman LR, Koduru S. Chemicals in the environment and developmental toxicity to children: a public health and policy perspective. Environmental Health Perspectives. 108 Suppl 3:443–48, June 2000.

3. National Prospective Cohort Study. Center for Children's Health and the Environment (web site), 2001.

Appendix II

1. Minshew NJ, Goldstein G, Siegel DJ. Neuropsychologic functioning in autism: profile of a complex information processing disorder. Journal of the International Neuropsychological Society. 3(4):303–16, 1997.

2. McFadden SA. Phenotypic variation in xenobiotic metabolism and adverse environmental response: focus on sulfur-dependent detoxification pathways. Toxicology. 111(1–3):43–65, 1996.

3. Wadman SK, Duran M, Beemer FA, Cats BP, Johnson JL, Rajagopalan KV, Saudubray JM, Ogier H, Charpentier C, Berger R, et al. Absence of hepatic molybdenum cofactor: an inborn error of metabolism leading to a combined deficiency of sulphite oxidase and xanthine dehydrogenase. Journal of Inherited Metabolic Disease. 6 Suppl 1:78–83, 1983.

4. London EA, Etzel RA. The environment as an etiologic factor in autism: a new direction for research. Environmental Health Perspectives. 108 Suppl 3:401–4, 2000.

5. Edelson SB, Cantor DS. Autism: xenobiotic influences. Toxicology & Industrial Health. 14(4):553–63, 1998.

6. NIEHS working group. A research-oriented framework for risk assessment and prevention of children's exposure to environmental toxicants. Environmental Health Perspectives. 107(6):510, 1999.

7. Nanson JL. Autism in fetal alcohol syndrome: a report of six cases. Alcoholism: Clinical & Experimental Research. 16(3):558–65, 1992.

8. Harris SR, MacKay LL, Osborn JA. Autistic behaviors in offspring of mothers abusing alcohol and other drugs: a series of case reports. Alcoholism: Clinical & Experimental Research. 19(3):660–65, 1995.

9. Aronson M, Hagberg B, Gillberg C. Attention deficits and autistic spectrum problems in children exposed to alcohol during gestation: a follow-up study. Developmental Medicine & Child Neurology. 39(9):583–87, 1997.

10. Rice D, Barone S. Critical periods of vulnerability for the developing nervous system: evidence from humans and animal models. Environmental Health Perspectives. 108 Suppl 3:511–33, 2000.

11. Ibid.

12. Goldman LK, Koduru S. Chemicals in the environment and developmental toxicity to children: a public health and policy perspective. Environmental Health Perspectives. 108 Suppl 3:443–48, 2000.

13. Myers GJ, Davidson PW. Prenatal methylmercury exposure and children: neurologic, developmental, and behavioral research. Environmental Health Perspectives. 106 Suppl 3:841–47, 1998.

14. Baraldi M, Zanoli P, Rossi T, Borella P, Caselgrandi E, Petraglia F. Neuro-behavioral and neurochemical abnormalities of pre- and postnatally lead-

exposed rats: zinc, copper and calcium status. Neurobehavioral Toxicology & Teratology. 7(5):499–509, 1985.

15. Ernst M, Moolchan ET, Robinson ML. Behavioral and neural consequences of prenatal exposure to nicotine. Journal of the American Academy of Child & Adolescent Psychiatry. 40(6):630–41, 2001.

16. Nulman I, Rovet J, Greenbaum R, Loebstein M, Wolpin J, Pace-Asciak P, Koren G. Neurodevelopment of adopted children exposed in utero to cocaine: the Toronto Adoption Study. Clinical & Investigative Medicine— Medecine Clinique et Experimentale. 24(3):129–37, 2001.

17. Budden SS. Intrauterine exposure to drugs and alcohol: how do the children fare? Medscape Women's Health. 1(10):6, 1996.

18. Goldman LK, Koduru S. Chemicals in the environment and developmental toxicity to children: a public health and policy perspective. Environmental Health Perspectives. 108 Suppl 3:443–48, 2000.

19. Liu G, Elsner J. Review of the multiple chemical exposure factors which may disturb human behavioral development. Sozial- und Praventivmedizin. 40(4):209–17, 1995.

20. Schantz SL. Developmental neurotoxicity of PCBs in humans: what do we know and where do we go from here? Neurotoxicology & Teratology. 18(3):217–27, 1996.

21. Bearer CF. The special and unique vulnerability of children to environmental hazards. NeuroToxicology 21(6):925–34, 2000.

22. Edelson SB, Cantor DS. Op cit.

23. Edelson SB. Unpublished manuscript. 2003.

24. Crinnion WJ. Environmental Medicine, Part 1: The human burden of environmental toxins and their common health effects. Alternative Medicine Reviews. 2000; 5(1):52–63, 2000.

25. Edelson SB, Cantor DS. Op cit.

Index